HANDBOOK FOR
PHYSICAL AND EMOTIONAL HEALING

HANDBOOK FOR

Physical and Emotional Healing

Cassandra Schamber, MD

Piedmont Publishing
Duluth, Minnesota

© 2011 Cassandra Schamber, MD. All rights reserved.

Published by:
Piedmont Publishing
2820 Piedmont Avenue, Suite A, Duluth, MN 55811
www.schamberhealing.com

Book design by Dorie McClelland, Spring Book Design

ISBN: 978-0-9832283-0-1
Library of Congress Control Number: 2011921509

For my mom

Contents

1 Introduction *1*

2 Energy *5*

3 Emotions *25*

4 The Intellect *65*

5 Shame *115*

6 The Intuition *129*

7 Dramas *139*

8 Life Lessons and Archetypes *165*

9 Conclusion *209*

1 Introduction

There is an epidemic of pain and suffering in the world today. People are both physically and emotionally ill, and physicians seem to be just spinning their wheels trying to keep up. While Western medicine has amazing technology at its fingertips, it can't get to the root cause of many chronic diseases to actually heal them. Physicians try one drug or one surgery after another, hoping that the newest drug or procedure will be the magical cure. But often it isn't.

Neither is the answer something as simple as taking herbs or supplements or changing your diet or exercise regimen. And the answer isn't as easy as doing meditation or getting alternative medical treatments. While all these things are beneficial for your health and may give you short-term relief, like Western medicine, they are limited in their ability to heal chronic medical diseases.

To experience true healing, you will need to do more than work with your body. You will need to dig deeper and work with other areas of your inner self. Your energy flow, your emotions, and your unhealthy intellectual patterns will all need to be brought into balance. You will also need to resolve any inner conflicts you have regarding your relationships and any painful lessons that life has brought you.

The fact that healing requires much inner work explains why

Western medicine and other therapies are limited in their effectiveness. They can be effective for simple problems, but they can't get to the deeper issues. Ultimately you are the only one who can get to the deeper issues and heal yourself. You are the only one who can identify all the areas of your life that are out of balance and do the work to bring them into balance again. While the responsibility may feel daunting, it is also exciting to realize that you have the power to heal yourself.

The concepts you will need to understand in order to learn how to heal yourself are actually very simple. Sometimes they can be deceptively simple. The problem is that while the concepts are simple, the work can be very challenging. At times it will seem like the hardest work you have ever done. While you may be tempted to skip over the more painful work that needs to be done, be aware that to get to the root of your problems there are no shortcuts. You can't ignore some aspects of your inner work because they are difficult or uncomfortable.

The nice thing about this work is that while at times it can be difficult, most people start to see changes in their lives rather quickly. The changes might be small at first, but they grow with time. So while you may not heal everything overnight, the improvements you see along the way will reinforce the fact that you are on the right path.

Don't stop seeing your physician because you are doing the work in this book. Instead, do your inner work while you continue to get your other medical treatments. Recognize that while your physician has his or her job to do, you are an equal partner in the job of healing yourself. You are the only one who can get to the root of many of the problems that cause you to be sick. It may be unrealistic for you to expect to cure congenital diseases or highly advanced diseases, such as heart disease or cancer. However, by doing the work in this book, you may find that even with those incurable diseases, you will be able to have a sense of peace about the situation.

The people who are most successful at healing themselves using the concepts in this book are the ones who are diligent and give

INTRODUCTION

themselves time to do the work. Don't simply plan on reading this book once and having things change overnight. Throughout the book there are many exercises for you to do, and you should regularly give yourself time to work on them. Do the exercises that feel right for you. Then later on go through the book again and you will discover other exercises that are applicable. The work of healing yourself is like peeling an onion: there are many layers of your inner self that you will need to expose and work with. Give yourself time to understand all the different layers so you can truly heal them.

2 Energy

Usually when we think of healing, we focus on our physical bodies and what we need to do to fix them. Our culture teaches us that our existence begins and ends with our physical bodies. But is that really true? Of course our bodies are vitally important to us, but they are not the only dimension of our health that is important. In addition to our bodies, we have our minds and our emotions. We also have our energy flow.

For thousands of years, Eastern healers have appreciated that underlying our physical existence is a vital life force that flows through us and supports our physical health. Different cultures refer to this life force with different terms. Practitioners of traditional Chinese medicine call this life force *qi* (pronounced *chee*). In India, Ayurvedic practitioners refer to it as *prana*. Western cultures refer to this life force as *energy flow*.

This fundamental life force supports all of the functions in our bodies and acts similarly to an electrical current, giving us the energy to keep our appliances running, so to speak. This life force flows through our bodies at all times while we are alive. When we die it dissipates, and the body that remains is an empty shell. Think about a person you know who has died. As she was dying, her life force began to weaken. You could see her slowly change and become weaker and less energetic. Finally, when she died, her vital life force completely left her body and was gone. Her body simply lay there and had none of the energy it had possessed when she was alive.

Energy is constantly flowing through our bodies while we are alive. Some people think it comes from the sky, and some think it comes from the earth, but for our purposes, the source doesn't really matter. The important thing to know is that it is constantly flowing through our bodies. Energy comes into us, flows through us, and then flows out of us as we exchange it with our environment.

When your energy flows into your body, it acts as fuel to feed your physical body and your mind. The cells in your body use energy to support their metabolism and perform their normal functions. Your mind uses energy to fuel its thoughts. You use energy when you relate to other people and when you do your work. You constantly use your vital life-force energy as you live your life.

In a healthy person, the energy flows in a balanced way. The flow is continuous and unobstructed, just as water flows in a stream that is being fed by a spring and that smoothly meanders along its natural path. Healthy energy flow is well balanced, without blockages or leakages. When your energy is flowing in a well-balanced way, you feel energized and physically healthy.

Problems arise when your energy flow becomes unbalanced. The flow can become blocked, the same way that water in a stream would if it became blocked by a fallen log. This impedes the energy flow and causes stagnation. Or the energy system may develop a leak, diverting some of the energy out of the system, similar to a small stream branching off from the main stream. This leakage decreases the strength of the energy flow downstream.

Blocked or leaking energy flow causes an imbalance in the energy system. Because your energy system is the foundation for your health, this imbalance in the energy flow causes many physical and non-physical problems. When your energy is out of balance, you may find yourself becoming more accident prone or getting fatigued, anxious, or depressed. As the energy imbalance becomes more pronounced, it causes physical illness.

I learned to appreciate the concept of energy flow when I started practicing acupuncture. For thousands of years, acupuncture has been used as one of the treatment modalities in traditional Chinese medicine. Acupuncture theory postulates that energy flows through our bodies in invisible channels called *meridians*. When energy is flowing freely through the meridians, the body feels balanced and healthy. But if the energy flow becomes weak or stagnant, the result can be physical or emotional ill health. There are many environmental, emotional, and social factors that can cause an imbalance in energy flow, for example, an unhealthy living environment, the wrong diet, physical trauma, or emotional trauma.

Acupuncturists use fine needles to stimulate specific points along the energy meridians to restore the balance of a patient's energy flow. As the energy flow improves, the patient's symptoms improve. Although acupuncture is limited in its effectiveness in healing advanced diseases, such as cancer, it can achieve some rather amazing results for a wide variety of physical and emotional symptoms.

I had a patient with chronic low-back pain who is a good example of how acupuncture can affect energy flow and the physical body. This patient's low-back pain dramatically limited her life. When she wasn't working, she spent all her free time resting and dealing with her pain. She had tried many different pain medications and had received cortisone injections in her back, but nothing provided relief. She was depressed and hopeless about her future.

When my patient started acupuncture, she did not have great expectations for what it could accomplish. But after a few visits, things started to change for her. Her pain improved some, but the thing that changed most dramatically was her energy level. Acupuncture acted to jump-start her energy battery. She was able to be more active, and her life became much more fulfilling because she had the energy to do what she wanted. She still had some back pain, but it stopped being the center of her life, and she could live quite easily with it. Of course not every patient responds in this dramatic manner, but success with patients like this one has helped me appreciate the importance of energy flow and how it affects the physical body.

You will need to understand the concept of energy and appreciate how it flows through your body as you work on healing yourself. Some people have the ability to see energy in the form of colorful clouds, called *auras*, that encircle people's bodies. Other people can sense energy flow in a tactile way, with their hands. When they place their hands on or near their body or someone else's, they can feel a vibration or heat or pressure that lets them know what is happening with the energy flow.

Some people can see or feel centers of concentrated energy, called *chakras*. Chakras are vortices or whorls of energy located on the body's midline, starting at the base of the spine and extending to the top of the head. There are seven main chakras. The first is the root chakra, located at the base of the spine. The seventh is the crown chakra, located at the top of the head. The other five chakras are spread out between the root and crown chakras. Each chakra is represented by a different color of the rainbow, starting with red for the root chakra and ending with violet for the crown chakra.

Each chakra is related to the organs in the region of the body where the chakra is located. The health of the organs in that region depends on the energy balance in that chakra. For example, the fourth chakra is in the chest region, and this chakra correlates with the heart, lungs, upper spine, and breasts. The health of the organs in the chest depends on the energy balance in the fourth chakra. If the energy in the fourth chakra is out of balance, the result may be a heart attack or breast cancer. We need to have healthy energy flow through the chakras in order to be physically healthy.

Many people use energy-healing therapies to bring their energy flow into healthy balance. Acupuncture is a common energy-healing therapy, but it is not the only one. Energy healers frequently use their hands to work with their patients' energy systems. To do this, they may put their hands on their patients' bodies, but often they can do this without touching the physical body at all. This is because the energy field is not limited to the physical body. Some common therapies that involve this type of energy work include Reiki, Qigong, and therapeutic touch.

It would be nice to use a diagnostic test to evaluate energy flow, especially if you can't see or feel it. Unfortunately, at this time there is not any generally accepted way to measure energy flow with a test or a machine. A process called *Kirlian photography* takes pictures of auras and energy using a photo-processing technique that is different from regular photography. But this technique is controversial, and it is not generally accepted as being a valid measure of energy flow. Because accepted diagnostic tests for energy flow are lacking, it is not possible to go to your physician, tell her your energy feels stagnant, and ask her to give you your energy value.

Since you can't measure your energy with a machine, you may wonder how you can find out how it is flowing. If you can't see auras or sense energy flow with your hands, what can you do? Fortunately you don't need to be able to see or feel your energy flow to know what is happening with it. You can actually sense it very easily by paying attention to how your body feels. Your body is always giving you input on how your energy system is working. It is like a barometer that is constantly giving you energy measurements.

You will know that your energy is flowing in a healthy and balanced way if you feel physically healthy. It's as though your energy battery is charged and feeding your physical body with the juice it needs to function properly. Your muscles will be relaxed, and your breathing will be slow and relaxed. You won't have uncomfortable symptoms, such as pain or an upset stomach. All your organ systems will feel as though they are running properly. You will feel as though you have plenty of energy to do whatever you need to do.

You can also pay attention to what is going on in your mind. When your energy is flowing in a healthy way, you won't be worrying or thinking too much. You won't feel depressed. You will be able to sleep easily at night and wake up refreshed.

At the opposite end of the spectrum is stagnant, depleted energy. In this situation you may feel depressed, fatigued, or physically uncomfortable. Your muscles may feel tense and tight, and when you pay attention to your breathing, you may notice that you breathe shallowly and rapidly. You may experience a number of physical problems when your energy is out of balance, including gastrointestinal upset, menstrual irregularities, upper-respiratory infections, bladder infections, or physical pain. The physical pain may come in the form of headaches, back pain, joint pain, or other body aches. You may feel exhausted and irritable. You may catch yourself thinking, *I have no energy today.* You may find that your mind is racing and you can't stop worrying or obsessing. You may notice that you can't relax easily and that you don't sleep well at night.

By observing your body and your mind, you can tell very easily how your energy is flowing. You don't need to be able to see your energy to know what is happening with it. You can simply stop and observe yourself, and you will get an incredible amount of information about your energy health. Assume that your energy is flowing easily if you feel physically and mentally healthy. Assume that your energy is out of balance if you have any type of physical or mental ill health.

▶*EXERCISE: Spend a few minutes, two or three times a day, sitting or lying quietly and paying attention to how your body feels and how your energy is flowing. Take some slow, deep breaths, and bring your attention to yourself. Pay attention to the tightness of your muscles and to how you are breathing. Notice how fatigued or energized you feel. Pay attention to any pain or discomfort you have and to how your organ systems, such as your gastrointestinal tract, are working. Pay attention to your thoughts. Imagine what your energy flow looks like. Try to physically sense the strength of your energy flow and detect any imbalances in the system.*

In addition to doing this exercise regularly every day, do it whenever you're feeling out of sorts or in pain. Use this exercise as your personal diagnostic tool to figure out how your energy is flowing. Don't judge what you are feeling as good or bad, and don't worry about how you're going to fix it. Your purpose now is to start listening to the messages your body is giving you and to think about your health from this new perspective. Don't just see your health as starting and ending in your body, but start seeing how your underlying energy flow is directly affecting your physical body.

Energy Expenditures
Another important aspect of energy flow involves your energy expenditures. After your energy comes into your body, it doesn't just idly sit there. It is dynamic and constantly flowing. It flows into you, and you use it to fuel your body and your mind, and then it flows out of you again. This flow is continuous for as long as you are alive.

The way your energy flows when it leaves your system is not totally random. You have input on the direction it will go. You are constantly deciding how you will spend it. You decide whom you are going to share it with. You decide what activities you will spend it on. And you decide what thoughts and ideas you will put it into.

We all choose where we are going to spend our energy and to whom we are going to give it. We may not always realize how much control we have over our energy expenditures. But whether we realize it or not, we are all one hundred percent in control of where our energy will be spent. How and where you spend your energy are key issues in deciding the quality of your physical and emotional health.

What do we spend our energy on? We spend it on the basic jobs we do every day to take care of ourselves. We put a certain amount of it into buying food, cooking meals, and cleaning our homes. We spend some of it on bathing, dressing, and grooming ourselves. We spend it on our work. We put energy into all the small errands we do, such as taking out the garbage and getting the mail. When you start to look at an average day in your life, you will find that you can identify a number of things you regularly spend your energy on.

In addition to your normal daily routine, you have special occasions, such as parties or vacations, that require extra energy. Or you may have a stressful situation, such as moving to a new house or looking for a new job, that will require extra energy. If you adopt a pet, you will need to put a certain amount of energy into taking care of your pet. And if you have a baby, you are committing to a lifetime of energy expenditures on your child. Every activity you choose to do requires you to spend energy on it.

It is important to know where you choose to spend your energy. You may not have much choice about putting your energy into activities such as grooming yourself or cleaning your house. But you might not realize how many choices you actually have over your energy expenditures. You make many energy expenditures out of habit because the people you know spend their energy the same way. For example, if all your neighbors put Christmas lights on their houses, you may choose to put your energy into putting lights up as well. If your entire family plans to go on a vacation to Mexico, you may choose to put your energy into taking a vacation with them. You may not feel that you have much choice about spending your energy on these things, because everyone else is doing them too, but the choice is yours nonetheless.

In addition to the activities we do, we put a lot of our energy into our relationships with other people. We give people our energy whenever we talk to them and whenever we spend time with them. Other people share their energy with us as well. The energy exchange between two people can be very strong. Although you may not be able to see it, you can almost physically sense it at times.

Have you ever had the sensation that someone was watching you? And then when you turned around, you saw your friend and she said hello, and you realized that the sensation of being watched was real? It was as if your friend had sent a line of energy out to you, and you could feel it. This is an example of an energy exchange. Your friend was giving her energy to you, and when you turned around and talked to her, you gave your energy back to her. If you stop and pay attention, you will be able to feel how energy can be almost palpable when you are exchanging it with another person.

Anytime you are involved with another person, you are spending energy on that person. If you talk on the phone with a stranger from another country, you are putting energy out toward that stranger. If you are sitting across from someone on the bus and the two of you are looking at each other, you are exchanging energy with that person. If you are listening to someone at work give a presentation, you are putting your energy out toward the speaker. Whether your interaction is relaxed or intense, short-term or long-term, you put some of your energy into that interaction.

People often spend energy on relationships that come together without very much planning or effort. You interact with people at school or work or in other places where you spend a lot of time. You may like some of these people, but there may also be people you wouldn't want to spend time with if you had the choice. Whether you like these relationships or not, they seem to happen naturally, without an obvious decision on your part, because they are part of the bigger situation. It is important to realize that you are putting energy into these relationships. Even if you haven't chosen them and don't particularly enjoy them, you are still putting energy into them.

You probably give less energy to your relationships that are more casual, and you give more energy to your relationships with your closest friends and family members. You also give a lot of energy to the people you have conflicts with. You can end up spending more energy on your greatest rival than you spend on your best friend.

In addition to spending energy on activities and relationships, people spend a lot of energy on their thoughts. For example, if you make plans for the future, you spend energy on your plans. If you are trying to figure out how to make a change in some aspect of your life, you are spending energy as you analyze the situation and try to figure out what to do next. You also spend energy as you look back and remember the past. Maybe you had a traumatic experience and it continually haunts you. You spend energy on the process of remembering that experience.

It is important for you to start to recognize all the ways that you consciously or unconsciously decide to spend your energy. Look at how you spend your time. What activities do you do throughout the day? Who do you spend your time with? What thoughts do you put your energy into?

As you start to watch your energy expenditures, also pay attention to how you feel about them. Do you feel that your time is well spent on valuable endeavors, or at the end of the day, do you feel that your time was wasted? Look at your relationships, and pay attention to the energy you spend on them. Are you giving energy to people who take it and squander it without giving you any support in return? Do you notice that those people seem to suck the life out of you? When you spend time with them, do you end up feeling drained and exhausted? Compare those relationships to the ones that make you feel energized and supported.

Pay attention to how you feel about your other energy expenditures. Do you spend your energy doing things that make you bored and depressed, or do you spend it on activities that make you feel rejuvenated and energized? What kind of energy exchange is going on at your workplace? Do you feel that the energy you put into your job is worth what your employer pays you, or do you feel underpaid and underappreciated?

Pay attention to the energy you spend on the institutions you have a significant connection to. Government systems, school systems, and health-care systems are all institutions that you probably spend energy on. For example, if you are a parent who is worried about where your child's school district is spending its money, you are giving energy to the school district. If you are a patient who is trying to get your health-insurance company to pay for a medical procedure, you are giving your energy to the insurance company.

Your financial situation is another area of your life that can give you big clues about how you spend your energy. Money flow is one of the most powerful symbols of energy flow. Where you spend your money is where you spend your energy. Of course we all need to spend a certain amount of money on our basic needs, such as food and shelter. But think about the other things you choose to spend your money on. If you spend it on things you can't afford, you are putting out energy you can't afford to lose. On the other end of the spectrum, if you have plenty of money and you choose to hoard it instead of using it for healthy causes, you may be blocking your energy flow.

Once you have used your money to buy something, it takes energy to take care of it. If you buy furniture or knickknacks, you will spend energy finding places to put them and doing whatever is needed to take care of them. If you buy a computer, you will have to spend energy getting it hooked up to your printer and to the Internet. You will also have to spend energy figuring out how to fix it if it breaks down. Everything we own requires energy at some point. We spend energy buying things, we spend energy taking care of them, and we spend energy disposing of them.

Pay attention to how you feel about your money expenditures. Do you feel satisfied with the way you spend your money? Do you feel that your financial situation is healthy and balanced, or do you feel that you are wasting your money and energy on things that aren't healthy for you? Do you look at the things you have bought and realize that you don't need them or that you aren't getting joy from them?

Pay attention to the other reasons you spend money. Do you feel a sense of peer pressure, and do you buy certain things to fit in? Do you feel pressure to buy a particular type of car so you'll look more successful? Do you dress a certain way to maintain a specific image? If you spend your money to fit in with a certain group of people, you need to be aware that you are giving your energy to that group and what they stand for. Pay attention to the groups you give your money and energy to, and ask yourself if you feel that those expenditures are healthy for you.

When you start to identify all the places you put your energy, you will see that the list is huge. This wouldn't be an issue if we all had an unlimited amount of energy available to spend. The problem is that there is a limit to our energy. While we always have energy flowing through our bodies, we have only so much energy to spend on a daily basis. If our energy was unlimited, we would never get tired and we wouldn't need to stop and rest and sleep. We would be like the Energizer Bunny, and we'd keep going and going and going.

But even the Energizer Bunny needs to have his battery changed from time to time. And we also need to get our batteries recharged. Once we've used up our allotment of energy, we get fatigued; then we need to rest so our bodies and minds can recharge. You may go through times when you have seemingly endless energy, but later on you will need to take some time out to rest and recharge. If you don't rest, eventually your mind will get tired, your body will get fatigued, and you will start to get sick.

It can be easy to put your energy out without paying attention to where you are putting it. But since we have a limited energy supply to work with each day, we need to spend it wisely. A healthy way to think about your energy expenditures is to put a unit value on them. This will help you break down your energy expenditures in a practical way. Imagine that you have a certain number of energy units—say, one hundred—to spend each day. You spend energy on your activities, your relationships, and your thoughts. Maybe on a certain day, working at your job takes forty units, cooking and cleaning take ten units, spending time with your spouse takes thirty units, and planning for the party you are going to have this weekend takes the last twenty units.

Start paying attention to where you are putting your energy units every day. How well do you ration them throughout the day? Do you find that by three o'clock in the afternoon your energy is spent and you're exhausted? Where are you going to get the energy for the rest of the day? Are you going to borrow it from tomorrow? from next week? Will you need to sleep late on Saturday morning to repay your energy units? If you don't let yourself sleep late on Saturday, when will you allow yourself to catch up? If you don't allow yourself to rest, over time you'll get more out of balance energetically and physically. You'll start to get fatigued. The cells in your body won't have enough energy to fuel their activities. How are you going to stay healthy if your cells don't have enough energy to fuel them? Eventually your energy imbalance will make you physically sick.

The concept of energy expenditures is vital for healing. It is important that you pay close attention to where you are choosing to spend your energy. Only when you are aware of the imbalances in your energy expenditures can you make the changes necessary to bring them into balance again.

▶*EXERCISE: Look at your calendar of activities. Identify the activities you dread and the activities you look forward to. Pay attention to how different activities affect your energy flow. If there are changes you can easily make in your energy expenditures, make them.*

▶*EXERCISE: As you go about your day, let yourself feel your response to different situations. Are you excited? peaceful? energized? Or are you depressed? fatigued? Which situations exhaust you, and which situations give you energy?*

▶*EXERCISE: Pay attention to how you feel when you spend time with other people. Are you excited and engaged? Or do you wish you weren't there, and do you find your mind wandering when you are with them? How are your interactions with other people affecting your energy flow? Do they energize you? Or do they suck the life out of you?*

▶EXERCISE: Look at your checkbook and credit-card statements, and pay attention to your money expenditures. Do you make healthy money expenditures? Or do you feel that your money would be better spent elsewhere? Remember that money is a physical manifestation of energy flow. Do you feel that your money choices support healthy energy flow?

▶EXERCISE: Pay attention to your belongings, and be aware of the energy you spend on them. Pay attention to how your energy feels when you are in your home. Is your home comfortable and easy for you to move around in? Or is it cluttered and filled with things that take your energy? If you find that you are spending too much energy on obtaining and caring for possessions, start to identify ways you can decrease those expenditures.

▶EXERCISE: Pay attention to where you spend your one hundred energy units every day. Look at your activities and relationships, and give them a numerical value that represents how much energy they require. Also be aware of how many energy units your thoughts are taking. Pay attention to whether you ration your one hundred energy units in a healthy way each day. And pay attention to whether you allow yourself to rest and pay back your energy bank when it gets depleted. Do you let yourself sleep late on Saturday when you are feeling fatigued? Or do you keep pushing yourself when your body is begging you for a rest?

▶EXERCISE: Imagine that each of your energy units is attached to a string, and watch how you send each string out to its allotted activity, person, or thought. For example, one string may go out to your toothbrush while you brush your teeth in the morning; one string may go out to your son as you talk with him about your plans for the day; one string may fly off into space with your worries. Pay attention to the areas of your life where the strings are most concentrated.

Energy and Lifestyle Habits

You may have noticed that in addition to the energy from your life force, there are also physical things that give you energy. We get energy from the air we breathe. We get energy from food and water. The sun is energizing for most people. And although exercise may be tiring in the short run, having a fit body is energizing in the long run. In addition to those basics, we each have specific activities that we find enjoyable and energizing, including our hobbies and socializing.

The way you treat your body is vitally important to your energy flow. You need to give your body what it needs to optimize that flow. Most people are aware that they need to take care of their bodies in order to be healthy. They know they should eat a healthy diet and exercise regularly. Unfortunately, it can be easy to develop unhealthy habits, and because of this, many people end up not taking care of their bodies the way they should.

As time passes, they start to realize that their unhealthy habits are taking a toll on their bodies. They realize that they need to take better care of themselves again. If they are overweight, they try different diets and exercise regimens, hoping they will find one that will work. If they have an unhealthy habit, such as smoking, they try to stop it. The problem is that they often have trouble following through and making the changes permanent. Why is it so difficult to make lasting lifestyle changes?

The answer comes down to energy units. If you really want to change your life, you will need to apply your energy to the change. Some habits don't require much energy for you to change them. For example, if you want to do something simple, such as adding a serving of fruit to your diet every day, you will find that it won't be very hard to do. It may require only three energy units every day for you to remember to get an orange out of the refrigerator, peel it, and eat it.

But what if you want to stop smoking? You may use forty energy units every day to stop yourself from taking a puff, and on bad days you may need to spend even more. You will need to put energy into not lighting up when you drink your coffee in the morning. You will need to put energy into not buying another pack of cigarettes when you go to the store. You will need to put energy into not smoking in every situation where you previously would have smoked. In the beginning you may need to spend eighty energy units every day to kick the habit.

The problem is that most people don't have an extra forty or eighty energy units to spend every day. Most people are functioning with a chronic energy deficit. How can you find an extra forty units if you are hundreds of units low? As much as you'd like to change your habits, if you don't have the energy to put toward the changes, you won't be able to follow through with them. This is why so many people find that they can't sustain their new diets or exercise regimens for more than a few weeks or months. For a while they borrow some extra energy units to apply to the changes. But eventually they need those units elsewhere, and they go back to their old ways.

Try a new approach if you are serious about changing your lifestyle habits. Don't force yourself to change things when you don't have the energy to follow through and make the changes permanent. Instead, let the surface details of the habits that you want to change wait for a little while. Do the work in this book and get your energy flowing in a more balanced way. As your energy flow improves, you will find that you have more energy units to apply to your lifestyle changes. You will then be able to make those changes permanent.

▶*EXERCISE: Look at the things in the physical world that give you energy. What foods and beverages make your body feel the most energized? What exercises make you feel the healthiest? What other things are energizing for you?*

▶*EXERCISE: Identify lifestyle changes you would like to make. If you have the energy to make your lifestyle changes, go ahead and make them now. But if you don't have enough energy units available, let the changes sit on the back burner. Take some time to work on bringing your energy flow into better balance. Then when you have more energy units available, you can start making the lifestyle changes.*

Energy and Chronic Pain and Chronic Diseases
Your body is affected when your energy flow is out of balance. Energy fuels our cells and supports their basic functions. Your cells will start to work less efficiently if your energy is not flowing in an optimal way. Over time the changes in your cells will become more entrenched and more problematic. You may initially have minor physical problems that are easy to resolve, but as your energy imbalance progresses, you will find that your physical problems become more difficult to heal.

The situation in which patients develop chronic pain is a good example of how an imbalance in your energy system can affect your physical health. As a pain specialist, I see a common theme among patients with chronic pain. I have many patients who are relatively young and have medical problems such as fibromyalgia syndrome and chronic headaches. Their pain can be devastating. Many of them stop working, and some end up spending most of their time resting in bed. They can't maintain their normal relationships because of their lack of energy. They often become isolated and depressed.

When I ask what these patients' lives were like before they got sick, many of them tell me how busy and active they used to be. Many of them were working mothers who would work long hours at their jobs every day and then go home to take care of their husbands and children at night. They had so many responsibilities at work and at home that they never had time to rest. They would go on, for years at a time, being sleep deprived and feeling guilty if they even considered stopping and resting. In addition to taking care of all their other responsibilities, many of them would push themselves to do extra things like volunteering and running marathons.

Then things would change. Some patients would start to have occasional body aches or headaches that would gradually worsen over time.

The pain would slowly become more intense and more constant until it caused them to stop doing almost all their normal activities. For other patients, the onset of the pain was shockingly sudden. They would be feeling fine one day, and the next day they would have a work injury or a car accident that would change their lives forever. They would become incapacitated almost overnight. In the end, whether their pain came on gradually or suddenly, all these previously highly functioning people become debilitated and could barely get out of bed.

Look at these patients' lives from an energy perspective. Before they got sick, they continually pushed themselves beyond the limits of what their energy systems could support. If you imagine that we each have one hundred energy units to use every day, you can see that these patients were probably using two hundred to three hundred units per day. Instead of stopping and resting regularly so their energy systems could rejuvenate, they would keep pushing themselves to work harder. Over time their energy systems became so out of balance that their physical systems couldn't sustain their lifestyles any longer.

Visualize the cells in the human body, and think about how they require energy to metabolize and function correctly. Imagine what happens to them if they are chronically being denied their vital energy. They end up responding like plants that don't get enough water. They get sick and stop functioning. It's no wonder that people who allow their energy to be chronically out of balance and depleted eventually become physically ill.

The example of relatively young patients developing chronic pain is a rather dramatic one, but the same concept applies to patients of all ages with chronic pain or other chronic diseases. Maybe your energy imbalance hasn't been as dramatic as this example. Or maybe your physical constitution is one that has allowed you to live in a state of energy imbalance for a longer time before you got sick. Or maybe you've been able to control your symptoms for some time before the energy imbalance became too severe. The age at which you get sick and your specific disease don't change the basic concept:

an imbalance in your energy flow leads to physical disease. If you have lived in a situation that has allowed your energy to become unbalanced, you are going to have to work on bringing it into balance again in order to heal yourself.

There are a number of things you can do to bring your energy flow back into balance. If you are exhausted, you may need to rest and give your body time to heal. Western medicine and alternative treatments can also be helpful.

But rest and medical treatments often aren't enough. You might feel better for a short time, but if your illness is caused by lifestyle habits that are unhealthy for your energy flow, resting or receiving medical treatments won't help forever. Over time the improvement you get from those treatments will be lost, and your energy imbalance will become obvious once again. This will cause you to be in a continual cycle of ups and downs, feeling better for a short while, but feeling worse again later on.

The purpose of this book is to help you bring your energy into healthy balance in a way that will be long term and sustainable. You will find that your improvement resulting from this work will be more enduring than the improvement you have gotten from medical treatments. You won't have the dramatic cycles of ups and downs commonly experienced with those treatments. It may take longer for you to feel better than you would with those treatments, but your improvement will be more stable and long lasting. You will be able to make your lifestyle changes permanent.

3 Emotions

Your energy needs to be flowing in a healthy way for you to have physical health. The big question is how can you bring your energy flow into healthy balance? Resting and receiving medical treatments may help, but that is not enough. There is a much deeper issue that needs to be addressed in order for you to bring your energy flow into balance. That deeper issue involves your emotions.

The connection between our emotions and our energy flow is profound. There is a direct correlation between our emotional flow and the quality of our energy flow. When our emotions are flowing in a healthy way, our energy is also able to flow in a healthy way. If our emotional flow becomes blocked, our energy flow will also become blocked. Our emotional system needs to be running smoothly in order for our energy system to be in balance.

We are all born with our energy flowing in a healthy, balanced way. Think about the children you know and their incredible energy levels. They run around and bounce and jump, and they are curious and engaged in life. They have so much energy that it can be exhausting for adults to keep up with them. Children are also born feeling their emotions in a healthy way. They may laugh hysterically one minute, and the next minute they may cry in agony when they fall and bump their knees. They can become paralyzed when they are afraid or can have tantrums when they are angry.

Children live in the moment. They don't think a lot about yesterday, and they don't spend much time planning for tomorrow. They experience each moment fully, in a way that most adults can barely remember. When children feel an emotion, it comes through them and they let it out without controlling it. They don't stop to wonder if their tantrums in the grocery store are going to embarrass their parents. They don't censor themselves or hold in their tears when everyone is staring at them. They aren't busy analyzing and judging themselves. They don't yet appreciate the rules that adults follow in order to be accepted in society. They don't really care if their behavior is considered appropriate or not. They just live the way their bodies tell them to live and feel the emotions their bodies need to feel.

Unfortunately, as children grow up, they learn from the adults around them to block their emotions. Adults have a good reason for teaching them to do this. They want their children to be accepted by other people, and they know that if their children continue to have dramatic displays of emotion, they won't fit in. Human beings are tribal animals, and we need our tribes to survive. Human babies aren't like reptiles. Their mothers can't just lay eggs and leave them to raise themselves. Babies can't go into the woods and find food and shelter on their own. They need their tribes to raise them and to teach them how to take care of themselves. They also need their tribes so they can socialize and enjoy other people's company.

It is important for children to learn how to deal with their emotions as they are learning to fit into their tribes. There would be chaos if all the members in a tribe were to go around feeling their emotions in the dramatic way that young children do. You can't have a meltdown every time things don't go your way. You can't lose your temper and become violent when you feel angry. If that were the case, the world would be chaotic and out of control. It would be like living in the Wild West, with people having gunfights whenever they were having a bad day.

As adults, we recognize that we all need to manage our emotions in order to fit into our tribes. Unfortunately, adults don't teach their children to do this in a healthy way. In an ideal world, children would learn to let their emotions continue flowing as they grow up. Adults would teach them that it is healthy to feel emotions of all types. But they would be taught to do this in a responsible way. They would be taught to not let their emotions cause them to create dramas or to hurt themselves or others.

Instead, adults teach their children a different approach to dealing with emotions. It is an all-or-nothing approach that teaches children that emotions are dangerous and need to be controlled. Children learn that they can either lose control and cry, scream, and create chaos or suppress all emotions and act stoically and do their work. There is no middle ground, no healthy way to both feel their emotions and function normally.

This approach gets passed down from one generation to another. Parents teach their children to block their emotions. When the children grow up, they teach their children to block their emotions, and so on. This has gone on for so long that it has become the accepted way to deal with emotions. It has become so automatic that people don't even realize there is another way to do it.

Even cultures that have the reputation of being more emotional foster this habit of blocking emotions. People in those more emotional, dramatic cultures may seem as though they are feeling their emotions in a healthy way, but often they aren't. They still block their emotions and allow them to build to unhealthy levels. The difference is that when their emotions build up, they've learned to decompress them by crying or yelling or making dramas. Their approach may be different from the more self-contained approach taken by more stoical cultures, but they are also using the all-or-nothing approach of dealing with their emotions. Their way simply looks different on the surface.

The all-or-nothing approach to handling emotions is very unhealthy. Emotions are physical, and they flow through our bodies.

Because they come from our bodies, there is a natural physical drive to let them flow. If you try to stop them from flowing, you have to work very hard to fight against your body's natural way of functioning. On a physical level, when you suppress your emotions you tighten up your muscles and tense up your body. This leads to physical pain and other uncomfortable physical symptoms. On a deeper level, when you block your emotional flow you block your energy flow, and this also leads to illness.

Even though suppressing emotions is not healthy, all children learn to do it. As they are growing up, they learn from the adults around them that they need to control their emotions in order to fit into their tribes. Emotional control can be very difficult for children because they are born being such emotionally spontaneous beings. They can have much inner conflict as they are taught to cut off the emotions and spontaneity that make their lives interesting.

The process of suppressing emotions is experienced differently by different children. They all have individual personalities, and they have different experiences within their tribes that affect how they will handle the suppression. Some children are able to cut off their emotional flow very easily, and the adults around them tend to approve of them because they are easy children to deal with. Some children find it more difficult to block their emotions, and they need continual reinforcement to remind them to stop feeling things so deeply. Those children may seem more dramatic and emotional than others, and they may have more conflicts with adults as they fight to maintain their natural way of being.

Some children block their emotions at such a young age that later, as adults, they can't remember ever feeling any emotions at all. Other children slowly learn to suppress their emotions in a stepwise process. They may learn early on to suppress one specific emotion, but they will continue feeling the others. With time they will also learn how to suppress the other emotions. For example, they may start suppressing their anger when they are told how bad it is to get mad, but they will still feel sadness and fear. Then as they get older, they will eventually learn how to block the sadness and fear as well.

Some children continue to feel their emotions for a long time, and then almost overnight they decide to block them. They may be exhausted from the pressure from the adults around them. Or they may decide that feeling emotions doesn't help them change their situation, so why keep feeling them. For whatever reason, they have a moment when they consciously decide to stop feeling their emotions. Later on, they can look back and remember a specific moment in their childhood when they decided that feeling their sadness or their anger was just too difficult and they were not going to do it any more.

The process of blocking your emotions cuts you off from your inner reality and your inner truth. While some children may appear to tolerate the process of blocking their emotions rather easily, most children experience a deep sense of loss and even a sense of trauma as they learn to ignore their inner reality. This loss can cause children to develop behavioral problems and physical symptoms. These symptoms are the first signs of the energy imbalance that comes with blocked emotions.

It is important to recognize that parents don't teach children to block their emotions out of a sense of cruelty, but more out of a sense of ingrained habit. So children in happy homes with the most loving and caring parents will learn this lesson just as strongly as children in abusive homes will. The children in the abusive homes may be more traumatized as they are being taught to block their emotions, but this lesson is universal, and it is not unique to abusive families.

The Emotional Organ
Imagine that you have an invisible organ inside your body called the *emotional organ*. This emotional organ is similar to your heart and lungs from the standpoint that it has a function to perform. Your heart has to beat, your lungs have to breathe, and your emotional organ has to allow your emotions to flow through it. Imagine a wide

cylinder that starts at the base of your spine and runs up through your body and out your head. Imagine your emotions as they come from deep inside you and work their way up and out of the cylinder. Emotions commonly come from deep inside us and flow out through our upper torsos and our heads. You may have a sense of butterflies or nausea in your abdomen and then laugh or cry as you release your emotions through your upper body.

There is a lot of confusion about emotions. People tend to think that emotions are felt in the mind and that they need to be figured out and analyzed in order to feel them. But actually you don't need to use your mind at all to feel emotions. The flow of your emotions occurs in your body and is a purely physical experience. Your body is born knowing how to feel them. Analyzing your emotional organ is like analyzing your heartbeat. Your mind doesn't need to analyze your heart for it to function in a healthy way; neither does it need to constantly analyze your emotional organ for you to feel your emotions in a healthy way.

The flow of emotions through your emotional organ is a physical process, just like breathing air or digesting food. As your emotions flow through your body, you can feel physical symptoms, such as tears or the pounding of your heart. Your emotional organ cannot be seen with your eyes the way your lungs and heart can be seen, yet it is just as important. If it is not allowed to function properly, you will eventually become sick, just as you would if you couldn't breathe healthy air or digest your food properly.

There are four key emotions that you need to let flow through your emotional organ: sadness, anger, fear, and joy. You have to let these emotions flow through you whenever they need to. You can't block them or try to change them. Your body knows how to feel these emotions in a healthy way, and you need to let them flow in the way that feels right for your body. There are two emotions that your body feels that aren't healthy: depression and shame. Feeling these emotions is not healthy for your energy flow. I'll discuss them later in this book.

The process of feeling emotions should be spontaneous and

unobstructed, just as your breathing is. Unfortunately, most people react in an unhealthy way when they start to feel an emotion. Instead of letting it flow, they get busy trying to figure out where it came from, if it's good or bad, and how to suppress it. Starting in their childhoods, they've learned to block their emotions, analyze them, and attach stories to them. An unhealthy reaction might be: *This emotion is anger, and I have to figure out where it came from. I think it came from the situation at work this morning when my jerk of a boss criticized my report.*

Now you will want to change the way that you deal with your emotions. You will want to focus on the purely physical aspect of the emotions, and put aside the analyses and stories you've attached to those emotions. If you are angry at your jerk of a boss, you will want to feel the physical feeling of anger rather than analyze it with your mind. Your goal is to learn how to feel your emotions again until you are as proficient at feeling them as you were when you were a young child.

Of course there are situations that need to be dealt with when they trigger your emotions. Feeling your emotions while staying in an unhealthy situation won't be beneficial for you in the long run. I'll discuss the details of how to manage such situations later, but the first step in changing those situations is to let your emotions flow again.

As you start to feel your emotions again, focus less on what caused them and more on the emotions themselves. The important thing is to feel the emotions that need to come through your emotional organ without judging them. This process is incredibly simple and basic. If we are all born doing it, it must not be that complicated. Little children don't sit around analyzing why a clown makes them so happy. They just accept their joy and laugh. If something makes them sad, they don't try to figure out why they are feeling sad. Instead, they just cry. They naturally know how to feel their emotions.

There are a lot of different words used to describe emotions. It may seem that simplifying the many emotions that we talk about into four key emotions is too simple. But most emotions are really just variations of the main four. For example, melancholy, sorrow, and inconsolable grief describe sadness. The intensity of sadness between melancholy and inconsolable grief may be different, but the body has the same type of physical sensation with both of them. Crankiness, irritability, bitterness, rage, and fury describe anger. The anger may be of different severities depending on which word you use, but it is still physically felt as anger. Apprehension, fright, and terror describe different levels of fear. Happiness, contentment, delight, and bliss describe different intensities of joy.

Most of the time that we spend feeling emotions is spent feeling one of the four key emotions. These are not the only emotions that people feel, but they are the four that get the most play time in the emotional organ. It is fine if you feel emotions other than the main four. You don't need to analyze them all and figure out every single emotion that can be felt. That would just be an exercise for your intellect, and it would defeat the purpose of letting your emotions flow.

Sometimes you may be feeling many emotions at once and not know exactly which ones you are feeling. That is fine. You don't need to analyze them, pick them apart, and limit yourself to feeling only one emotion at a time. Whatever needs to come through your emotional organ will come through when the time is right. It is your job to let that happen. The important thing to remember is that the process of feeling emotions should be spontaneous and should not be controlled. Whatever needs to flow should be allowed to flow. If you are angry all day, every day for six months, you need to feel angry for six months. If you are joyful one minute and sad the next, you need to let your joy and then your sadness flow for as long as they have to.

When you are trying to identify your emotions, you may need to put some effort into remembering what they feel like. If you are like most people, you've learned to almost completely block at least one key emotion and maybe two, three, or even all four. It is your job to learn again what it feels like to physically feel them. While everyone can feel different physical sensations as they feel their emotions, there are some common sensations that most people experience. Joy is usually felt as a lightness of being and exuberance, and you will probably find yourself smiling and laughing. Sadness is usually experienced as a sense of longing in your body, and most people cry when they are sad. Anger is a difficult emotion to feel because people tend to either suppress it or project it toward other people. Healthy anger may be experienced as an irritable physical intensity with rapid breathing. Fear is frequently felt with a racing heart, rapid breathing, nausea, sweating, and shaking. If you breathe very rapidly because of your fear, you may also feel light-headedness and tingling in your hands and around your mouth.

As you feel your emotions, you may have different physical sensations than those mentioned here. Your goal is to get to know your own body and be able to know what all four key emotions feel like as they come through your emotional organ. You may not be able to recognize all four when you start this process. Or maybe you will be able to recognize all four, but you may have trouble letting them flow easily. It can take time to be able to both recognize them and allow them to flow without suppressing them.

When you are feeling your emotions, you will want to be able to let them flow as easily as they did when you were a young child. You will want them to flow spontaneously, feeling whatever needs to be felt whenever it needs to be felt. The amount of time you spend feeling each emotion cannot be judged.

Sometimes you may have a specific situation that triggers your emotions. At other times you may feel an emotion and not know why. You may wake up in the morning feeling sad or angry and not know what caused you to feel that way. Your goal will be to feel that emotion, no matter what you suspect the cause to be. If something or someone triggers an emotion for you, set aside the cause and feel your feelings. You can deal with the cause of your emotions later. The most important thing at this point is to focus on feeling your emotions as fully as possible.

The process of allowing your emotions to flow spontaneously can be difficult at first. This is because we get taught to control and suppress them from the time we are young. Many people only allow their emotions to flow occasionally, for example, during times of intense stress. For example, if someone close to you dies, you may allow yourself to feel intense emotions in response to their death. But society says that you shouldn't grieve for too long, so even if you are not done feeling your emotions, you try to leave the grief behind and return to the habit of suppressing your emotions again.

Most of us have one or two emotions that we have personally decided are acceptable for us to feel. We channel all our other emotions into the one or two that are acceptable. For example, if you only let yourself feel sadness, you will cry not only when you are sad but also when you are afraid and angry and happy. Because you aren't comfortable feeling the other emotions, you may end up crying whenever any of the other emotions start to come through you.

We don't just casually choose which emotions we'll decide are acceptable to feel. The choice isn't usually conscious at all. Instead, we learn what is acceptable to feel from our culture and from the people around us. Our family, friends, and communities are constantly giving us input into what we should feel. For example, if the people in your family all cry very easily, you may feel comfortable crying.

Our religious and ethnic communities give us input on which emotions are acceptable to feel and how to feel them. In some religions, people sing and shout with joy, while in others, people are much more self-contained. The same thing happens with different ethnic groups. Some ethnic groups find it acceptable to express joy or sadness, while others frown upon any outward expression of emotion at all.

Gender stereotypes are powerful in telling us which emotions we should feel. In the past, women were stereotypically taught that anger was a bad emotion to feel. It was considered very unfeminine and unbecoming. On the other hand, women were taught that sadness was acceptable for them to feel. So when women were angry, they often ended up crying because they were more comfortable feeling sadness than anger. Many women today still have trouble feeling their anger. "I was so mad, I cried" is a common phrase that many women still find themselves saying. Interestingly, with the relatively recent entrance of women into the male-dominated workplace, anger is becoming more accepted and even respected in women. Now many younger women feel anger more easily than they feel sadness.

Men have stereotypically been taught that sadness is a bad emotion to feel and that sadness is a sign of weakness. "Boys don't cry" has been an anthem for men all over the world. Currently we are starting to accept the idea that men can feel some sadness, but we are still somewhat ambivalent about seeing men cry. We still aren't sure if we are comfortable knowing that strong men can feel vulnerable emotions.

The emotion that is most acceptable for men to feel is anger. Men learn that whenever they are sad or afraid, they had better feel anger instead so they can look tough. It must be noted that the anger many men feel and express by yelling, screaming, or having tantrums, is not a healthy way to experience anger. Feeling anger in this way is just as unhealthy as feeling nothing at all.

Fear is an emotion that is unacceptable for men *and* women. There is a real stigma associated with feeling fear. We have been taught to judge fear as an indication of being vulnerable, weak, and pathetic (and who wants to be vulnerable, weak, and pathetic?), so we do our best to block our fear, and we may become angry or sad instead.

All human beings feel fear, whether they've ever admitted it to themselves or not. To be human is to experience the fear of the unknown. We all have times when we don't know what the outcome of a situation will be. For example, you may have a child who is sick or wonder whether your spouse is going to leave you or worry about finances. And finally, there is the ultimate fear: the fear of death. Will it be painful? Where do we go after we die? Will there really be a heaven or will we disintegrate?

There are always new issues coming up that force us to face the unknown future. These issues trigger fear. Unfortunately, we get taught to suppress our fear. We are told that if we have fear, we don't have faith in God. We are also told that if we have fear, we won't succeed. These messages make it very hard to acknowledge and feel our fear.

Some people deal with their fear by channeling it into anger or sadness. They may explode in anger or cry inconsolably when they are feeling deep fear. They can also suppress their fear until their bodies can't hold it in anymore. When they suppress it, over time it can build up and put great pressure on the emotional organ. When the pressure is too great, the fear explodes out like a volcano, and it causes them to have intense physical symptoms, such as a panic attack or chest pain. Then as the intense fear moves through them, the physical sensations can make them think they are dying, and this escalates their fear even more. With practice fear can be felt in a way that isn't so stressful.

Joy can be a problematic emotion to feel in our culture because we have put limitations on where, when, and how much we should feel it. Our culture often pressures people to be in a good mood, but not in too good of a mood. Although we all want to feel joy, most of us censor our joy. Think of little children laughing uncontrollably when they are happy. Do you let yourself do that? Most people don't. And because they are so busy censoring themselves, they get annoyed when someone else is too happy.

Sometimes you may be feeling joy, but you block it because of a situation you are in. For example, most of the time people frown upon someone who seems too happy at a funeral. We have learned that funerals are a time of sadness, so you had better not laugh at a funeral. But maybe you are remembering the happy times you had with the deceased. Maybe you spent the last two days crying and now you feel a sense of joy. You can't judge the fact that you are feeling joy when everyone around you is sad.

Sometimes you may wish that you could be happy, but you just aren't. For example, during the Christmas season, you probably feel intense pressure to be happy. But if you just lost your job and are having financial problems, you may not be feeling much joy. Or maybe Christmas is the anniversary of your mother's death. The holiday may be reminding you of all the Christmases you had with her in the past. You may be feeling grief, and the last thing you want to do is smile. Our culture tends to tell us to suck it up and act happy even when we aren't. But it isn't natural or healthy to fake emotions just because everyone else is feeling them.

Emotions shouldn't be judged. It is important to accept whatever you are feeling and let the emotion flow through you, no matter what is happening around you and no matter what other people are feeling. You don't necessarily need to involve everyone else in your emotions. You can feel your joy quietly to yourself at the funeral, or you can feel your anger and sadness quietly to yourself at a Christmas party. But don't block one emotion and try to replace it with another. It is not healthy to block some emotions while letting others flow. This causes you to go against your body's natural way of doing things. It may seem okay to use the flow of your more accepted emotions to take the edge off your less desirable emotions. But when you do that, you are limiting the ability of your emotional organ to work most effectively.

Your objective is to have the emotional organ open twenty-four hours a day, seven days a week. You won't necessarily be feeling intense emotions that whole time, but you want your emotions to have access to come through your body whenever they need to. Sometimes you will find that you have an emotion that needs to flow for hours or days on end. Sometimes your emotions will come out all mixed together in an intense jumble. Sometimes you will be in neutral, and no emotions will need to flow. The important thing is that you let your emotions flow whenever they need to.

Positive and Negative Emotions
People commonly refer to joy as a positive emotion and to anger, sadness, and fear as negative emotions. We have learned to judge

emotions as good or bad depending on how comfortable we are with them. We like joy because it is a pleasurable emotion to feel and because our culture teaches us that it is a good emotion. We tend to dislike the other emotions because they make our bodies feel things we aren't so comfortable with. And we have learned that they are dangerous and that they will hurt us.

Because we have learned that the uncomfortable emotions are dangerous, we try to suppress them. But because feeling emotions is a natural body process, it is very hard to hold them in. If we don't allow them to flow in a healthy way, they can build up and might explode out of us in the form of rage or a panic attack. Or the suppressed emotions might come out in little spurts that cause us to make passive-aggressive comments that hurt other people in subtle ways. Or if we are able to totally hold our emotions in, they sit inside us like abscesses, using up all our energy units as we work to keep them from flowing.

It makes sense that you would consider negative emotions to be dangerous if you have been told your entire life how bad they are. It is also easy to consider them dangerous if you have learned to deal with them in a way that hurts yourself or others. But if you learn to feel them in a responsible, healthy way, they will lose the negative association. You will find that letting them flow is a relief and isn't anywhere near as dangerous as you thought it was.

Many books and articles have been written by psychologists, physicians, and researchers who insinuate that experiencing the negative emotions is potentially harmful to your health. That is not true. The problem is that few people really understand emotions, including the experts. Some experts approach emotions in an intellectual way, as if emotions were thoughts or actions. The research those experts do is flawed because they don't understand the basics of how emotions should be experienced. They may do research on anger and consider the emotion of anger to be the process of yelling at others. If their research shows that people who yell at others have a higher risk of heart disease, they conclude that it's dangerous to feel anger. But the process of feeling anger in a healthy way is a completely different experience from yelling at other people, and the two can't be compared.

Instead of viewing anger, sadness, and fear as negative emotions, see them in a different light. Think of them as uncomfortable rather than dangerous. This will make them seem less intimidating. Of course they are not always uncomfortable to feel, but there are times when they can give you physically uncomfortable sensations. For example, the physical intensity associated with anger can be uncomfortable, especially when it is strong. The symptoms of strong fear, such as a racing heart and light-headedness, can also be uncomfortable.

Different people will find some emotions to be more uncomfortable than others. For example, you may find that anger is not uncomfortable for you at all, but sadness is. Another person may find that fear is physically uncomfortable, but anger and sadness are no big deal. Although emotions may be uncomfortable at times, they are in no way dangerous, as long as you experience them responsibly and don't project them onto others or injure yourself while you are feeling them.

When we judge emotions as positive or negative, we learn that we should take a goal-oriented approach to feeling them. We are taught that the purpose of life is to be happy all the time and that there is something wrong with us if we aren't happy. Instead of opening our emotional organs up to whatever emotion needs to come through, we try to hold back our anger, sadness, and fear, and we let only joy come through. But it is unrealistic to expect that you can avoid feeling your uncomfortable emotions and only feel joy.

This unrealistic expectation can drive people to look for external ways to trigger joy. They think that if they aren't happy enough now, they may feel more joy once they've found the perfect relationship, the perfect job, the perfect house, or the perfect car. They think that they can avoid their uncomfortable emotions by continually acquiring new things or having new experiences. Of course we do feel joy when we acquire something we want, but that joy doesn't last forever. Today you may be ecstatic because you bought your dream car, but eventually that car will become your old car, and your joy may fade, just as the car's paint job does. And the uncomfortable emotions are still inside of you, waiting to come through your emotional organ.

No one emotion is better than any other. If emotions are felt in a healthy way, they are all equally valuable. Embrace all the emotions that flow through you, and you will find that your joy will be more intense and your other emotions will become just another part of you, instead of being something to avoid.

EMOTIONS BLACK-BOX WARNING

In the United States, when a drug has a potentially dangerous or harmful side effect, pharmaceutical companies include a black-box warning on the medication instructions to warn physicians of this dangerous side effect. There is one black-box warning you need to be aware of when you learn about the process of feeling your emotions, and it is very important that you never do this one thing. The black-box warning for this process is: **You must NEVER act out and hurt yourself or anyone else while you are feeling your emotions.**

If you are feeling anger and you are tempted to put your fist through the wall—don't. If you are mad at someone because he insulted you, don't say or do anything to him at all. You can deal with him later, after you have calmed down. The experience of letting your emotions flow is entirely a personal one. This means that your feelings are your own experience and no one else's business. Someone may trigger an emotion in you, but he is just an outside entity, and he has no part in your process of feeling that emotion. Every emotion is one hundred percent your own responsibility to deal with.

Emotions should never be projected onto other people. For example, anger should never be projected onto others through yelling or physical violence. Unfortunately, our culture teaches us that anger is an outwardly explosive emotion filled with hostility, aggression, yelling, and physical violence. That assumption is completely wrong, and those behaviors are not healthy displays of anger. You waste your energy and cause more misery for yourself when you project your emotions onto others.

Passive-aggressive behavior is another form of projected emotions, especially anger, and it should never be used. Passive-aggressive behavior consists of snotty, snide, and insulting comments or actions that aren't overtly aggressive but are meant to bite. For example, when you are mad at someone who you know is trying to lose weight, you may slip into the conversation the comment that her dress is looking a little tight. Passive-aggressive comments can be just as cruel as punching someone. Watch yourself, and if you find yourself making those types of remarks, you know you are projecting your anger.

You will need to be very careful when you feel anger, especially in the beginning. As you start to feel it, you will need to pay attention to the safety of yourself and others. It can be easy to let yourself get out of control when you are feeling anger. That is not acceptable. If you are worried in the beginning about losing control when you are feeling anger, go off by yourself and feel it by yourself, on your own time. Leave the people you are with, and go into another room where you can be alone. When you are alone, you can let your emotions flow without being tempted to involve other people in the process.

When you are feeling anger, avoid yelling and screaming because those actions are hard on your vocal cords. Punching things is obviously not a good idea; you don't want to hurt your hand or the thing you were going to punch. The only thing you can safely punch is a pillow. You could also try other safe physical activities, such as kneading bread or clay. Another way to release anger is by hitting your couch or bed with a sock roll. Make sure that whatever activity you do will not hurt you physically.

You may find that you want to do some type of physical exercise, such as running, to burn off your anger. That might work, but once again, be careful to maintain control of your body as your anger comes out. You don't want to risk harming your body because you are so angry that you aren't watching your footing while you run.

Another problem with using physical exercise as a mechanism to help you experience anger is that it may actually stop the flow of anger. For many people, exercising produces endorphins. The endorphins will make them start to feel happy. If this happens, the process of running isn't going to facilitate the healthy flow of anger. If you have anger to feel, you need to stop and let yourself feel it. Later, you can go running and feel happy.

Usually the safest way to feel anger is to sit in a chair or lie on a bed and let it flow without too much body movement so you won't be tempted to hurt yourself or someone else. That may be hard to do at first, but with time you'll get used to it. If you find that you tighten up your muscles and get physical pain in response to feeling your anger, you may need to do some type of safe movement to keep your muscles relaxed. Shaking your hands and waving your arms can help you keep your muscles loose while you feel your anger.

Another way to feel your anger without tightening up your muscles is to do labor-style breathing with a more rapid breath rate than is used in relaxation breathing. Try saying *whoo-whoo, whoo-whoo* as a guide when you are breathing out your anger. Slow down your breathing if you start to get light-headed; speed it up again when the light-headedness subsides.

Swearing can be a very effective way of helping you feel your anger. There is something about the combination of vowels and consonants in swearwords that can be very helpful at bringing the physical intensity of anger out through your body. Maybe the fact that swearwords are often forbidden also makes them desirable words to say when you are angry. If you are averse to saying swearwords, find an acceptable word that brings out the same physical intensity in your body and use it instead. You can use these words like a mantra, repeating them over and over again, quietly to yourself, to bring your anger out through your body.

Another dangerous projected emotion is fear. People start fights and nations start wars because of projected fear. When they come up against situations that are scary for them, people have a tendency to jump into action before they've felt their fear. They think that they will be safe if they take action. Of course you do need to make changes in your environment if it isn't safe, but if you are acting out of fear, it is easy to make unhealthy choices. Unfelt fear can make it hard to see the big picture. It can make you do things that you may later regret.

If you aren't used to feeling your fear, you may be uncomfortable when you first start to feel it. You may be tempted to take action to avoid feeling it, but this is not healthy. Fear is one of the four key emotions, and it can't be ignored. If it wants to come out, you need to feel it.

Unless you are in a dangerous situation that is immediately threatening your safety, you shouldn't rush into any action that you are tempted to take out of fear. It is much healthier to feel your fear first and act later when you are calmer. It is much more beneficial for your energy system if you approach your life this way. You will also find that with this approach, you won't need to create so many dramas that hurt yourself and others.

The Lid on the Emotional Organ

The intensity of your emotions can be especially strong when you first start feeling them. Imagine that your emotional organ has a lid or a floodgate on the top of it. The lid can be opened and closed as needed to adjust the intensity of the emotional flow. Most people keep the lids on their emotional organs tightly closed. They may occasionally allow the lids to open when the pressure of their emotions builds to excessively high levels. This relieves some of the intensity of the emotional pressure inside them, but then they think, *Oh, my goodness, feeling all these emotions is dangerous, so I'd better stop feeling them.* They close the lids and block their emotional flow again.

This is why so many people's emotional experiences feel so out of control to them. When you don't allow your emotions to flow the way your body would like them to, pressure builds up inside your emotional organ like an abscess filling with pus. With time the pressure gets too great, the lid on the emotional organ is forced open, and the emotions spew out.

People can get intensely emotional in response to seemingly minor emotional triggers. This is because their emotional organs are in a constant state of overload, like abscesses waiting to explode. Even the smallest triggers have enough power to force the lids open and cause the emotions to flood out. You might normally be the most cheerful person in the world, but every once in a while you might have a bad day and end up crying hysterically over a little thing like getting a run in your pantyhose. Or you may get out of control and yell at your kids over something stupid that you will later regret. That lack of control is because you have allowed the pressure in your emotional organ to build to a level that is too high to sustain. You then need to use minor irritations to open the lid and relieve some of the pressure.

Most people live in states of constant emotional overload. They don't know how to open the lids on their emotional organs to let their emotions flow in a healthy way. It makes sense that when you have been taught your entire life to block your emotions, you would have trouble allowing the lid to open easily. So instead of simply allowing your emotions to flow on a regular basis, the emotional pressure builds and you end up needing to use whatever outside situation is available to open the lid and get the emotions flowing. You may be in a situation that wouldn't normally upset you, but because the pressure in your emotional organ has built up so much, you use the seemingly minor trigger to open the lid and release the pent-up pressure.

You need to understand how the emotional organ works as you start this process of learning how to feel your emotions again. If you've spent your entire life trying to keep the lid on your emotional organ closed, you probably have quite a bit of emotional pressure built up. Now you might be thinking that you'll open the lid just a tiny crack to see what feeling emotions is all about. However, instead of opening up just a tiny crack, the lid could fly open, like a floodgate, from the pressure of years of pent-up emotions, and the intense emotions will come spewing out.

When you open the lid on the emotional organ, your body is so thrilled to rid itself of the abscessed emotions that it can get very enthusiastic about releasing them. This is especially true with fear. You may find yourself breathing so rapidly with fear that you start to have tingling in your hands or lips or feel light-headed. You might have such intense fear that you start to shake and feel as though you are having a panic attack. Your symptoms will get less dramatic as your emotional organ decompresses, but it can be intense and uncomfortable to feel these symptoms at first.

If the emotional flow is very intense in the beginning, remind yourself that feeling emotions is a healthy thing. While emotions may be uncomfortable, they are not dangerous. Remember that when the initial flood of emotions starts to smooth out, you will be able to handle it more easily. Give yourself time and energy units to spend on feeling your emotions. Let yourself stop and rest when they tire you out.

You may find that taking little breaks from feeling your emotions can help if you are very uncomfortable with their intensity. If you are feeling out of control with any emotion, pay attention to your breathing. It is common to breathe rapidly with intense emotions, especially with fear and anger. If you catch yourself hyperventilating, slow down your breathing for a while. Then after a short rest, let the lid open and let your emotions flow again.

If you have trouble slowing down your breathing, find someone to talk to, either on the telephone or in person. When we talk with other people, we usually suppress our emotions because our minds are busy analyzing our conversations. When you are talking to that other person, you will probably find yourself going back to your unemotional state. You don't have to tell them what is going on with you; just talk about the weather. You can also go for a walk or go shopping. Being in public can achieve the same effect as talking with someone. It diverts your attention and slows down your emotional flow. Take a break from feeling your emotions, and go back to feeling them again after you have rested.

It is common for people with intense fear go to their physicians or the emergency room for treatment. They may have been taught that fear is dangerous, and they may be afraid that something bad will happen to them when they start feeling it. If you go to the emergency room, the staff might conduct some tests and you might be given medication to help you relax. You may need to do this once to be reassured that feeling intense fear isn't harmful for your health. But as you get more comfortable with it, you won't need to go to the physician anymore.

It would be nice if you had a family member or friend with whom you could share this new concept of emotions. You could ask that person to sit with you as you start to feel your deep emotions, especially your fear. The two of you could also talk about the concepts in this book as a way to help you apply them to your lives. In a relatively short time, you will find that you will feel more safe about feeling your emotions, and you will be able to feel them without having someone by your side. As you start to experience what it feels like to let your emotional organ function in a normal, healthy way, you will get more comfortable with the whole idea of feeling emotions.

If you have had an intense emotional experience in the past, you may be worried about feeling that emotion again. You may have a history of panic attacks or of intense anger that led to you to do something to hurt someone. Or you may have had an intense grief experience that got labeled as a nervous breakdown. Although you may have had difficult emotional experiences in the past, that doesn't mean it is dangerous for you to feel those emotions again. When you have a different understanding of emotions and are focusing on feeling them in a healthy, responsible way, your experience with them will change. You will start to see them as a natural, healthy thing and not something you have to avoid.

Trust that the intensity of the emotional flow that can come in the beginning will stabilize with time and won't always be so intense. If you are especially uncomfortable with one specific emotion, do exercises to trigger the other emotions first and then go back and work with the uncomfortable one later on. For example, if you have a history of severe anxiety and panic attacks, work on triggering sadness and anger before returning to fear. The same concept applies to anger and sadness; if you are very uncomfortable feeling one of them, do exercises to trigger the other emotions first. If you have a history of becoming dramatic or violent when you feel anger, practice feeling your sadness and fear; you should find that as you learn to feel the other emotions, your anger won't be so intense. Eventually you will need to feel all four key emotions for the emotional organ to work in a healthy way. But you can start the process by getting used to the emotions that are more comfortable for you first.

The more effort that you put into this process, the sooner you will get results. But the process of feeling emotions can't be forced. Don't think that you can just sit by yourself in a room feeling your emotions for a year and then you'll be done. This is a change in lifestyle. As you practice feeling your emotions again, you will start to do it naturally and without thinking about it. It will become a way of life that feels right because you are coming back to the root of your human nature. As your emotions start to flow, you will get a sense of relief. Your body will be relieved to have the emotions flowing through it again, and your muscles will be able to relax. It is as though you are returning home to a secure place that has always been inside you, but that you forgot about. Another advantage is that as your emotional flow opens up, you will start to have increased energy. You won't need to put your energy units into keeping the lid on your emotional organ closed, and you will be able to use those extra units for other more regenerative endeavors.

Cleaning Out Your Emotional Basement

Most people spend their entire lives blocking their emotional flow. When you block your emotional flow, your emotions can't get out of your body in the healthy way they should. If you don't let them out of your body, they don't simply disappear; instead, they end up getting stuck inside you. Imagine that your inner self is like a house. In our houses we have closets and basements for storage. Our inner selves have the equivalents of closets and basements where we store all the emotions we have suppressed.

The process of storing our suppressed emotions starts when we are children. For example, maybe one day when you were a little child you were feeling fear, but your older brother told you not to be a sissy, so you put your fear into your inner hall closet. On another day, maybe your sister stole your toy and made you angry, but your mother told you it was wrong to get mad at your sister, so you put your anger into your inner hall closet and went back to playing. You continued to store unfelt emotions in your inner hall closet until it became full. Then you went on to fill all the closets inside you, and finally, you started to store your emotions in the basement.

Every time in your life that you have suppressed an emotion, you have stored it inside you. Now after many years of doing this, you can imagine walking through your inner basement and seeing all the rooms full of emotions. You can see the names of situations or people associated with those unfelt emotions written on the doors to those rooms.

We all have basements inside us that are full of suppressed emotions. As you start to feel your emotions again, you will need to do some serious housecleaning. Your body doesn't like to have all those emotions stored inside it. Those stored-up emotions cause pressure to build up in your emotional organ, and your body has to work hard to keep them from coming out.

Your body doesn't like to have to put so much of its energy into holding the lid on your emotional organ closed. When you decide to open the lid, even a little bit, your body will want to clean the basement. It will want to let all the stored emotions flow out. It will want to keep the lid open until your emotional basement is all cleaned out. You may not be thrilled about having to do this, but you need to do it to heal yourself.

You need to let yourself feel all your sadness, fear, and anger for as long as you need to. You can't judge the timing of your emotional flow. If you are doing this correctly, you will probably feel intense emotions for hours on end and for days or weeks at a time. Your goal is to be open and to allow all the emotions to flow out.

You may not always remember the details of the situations that originally caused the emotions you have stored in your emotional basement. Maybe you were too young to remember them, or maybe you were so effective at blocking your emotions that you did not recognize when situations triggered them. For example, maybe you stored fear in your emotional basement from a situation that occurred when you were twelve. Back then you put the fear in your emotional basement so you wouldn't look scared in front of your friends. Now several years later, your body has decided to clean out the fear. You don't necessarily need to remember the details of why you feel the fear. It is more important to feel the fear and release it from your body than to remember the story behind it.

The amount of time it takes to clean out the emotional basement is different for everyone. It commonly takes months to years. If you really want to get to the root of your physical and emotional problems, you can't skip this work. No one knows the length of time it will take for you. You may decide to feel your emotions for a little while and then decide that's all you want to do for now. You can always do more housecleaning later on. But you may find that once you open the lid on the emotional organ, your body is so relieved to rid itself of your abscessed emotions that it won't let you stop feeling them even if you want to.

If you stay committed to this process, you will eventually clean out your emotional basement. Your emotions will become less intense, and you will feel more inner peace. You may still have times of intense emotion, but these times will be less frequent and easier to deal with. You will also find that because you understand what is going on in your body, you won't be so shocked when the intense emotions come through you.

You will eventually find yourself being able to feel your emotions while you go about your daily life. You won't need to take time out to process them. For example, you may be talking with a coworker and getting angry about something she is saying. With experience, you will get to the point where you will be able to feel your anger while you are talking with her, and it won't get in the way of what you are doing. Your emotions will flow without obstruction, yet they won't need to be a hindrance to your activities.

How to Start Feeling Emotions
It may take some time in the beginning for you to figure out how to feel your emotions again. Ultimately you need to be able to feel all four healthy emotions: joy, sadness, anger, and fear. You need to be able to feel them physically as they come through your body. You need to be able to feel them spontaneously—day or night—whenever they are ready to come through you.

How do you start to feel your emotions? You may need to be somewhat deliberate about feeling them at first. Because feeling emotions has become such a foreign experience for so many people, it is something that frequently needs to be relearned. You may need to put in some time and effort to do this in the beginning. You may need to practice feeling your emotions with exercises, as though you are learning a new workout technique. With time it will become a habit, and you will do it naturally without needing to think about it.

Start by putting time aside to work on this every day or as often as you can. You don't have to have a rigid schedule, but the more time and effort you put into it, the sooner you'll get the hang of it. You may need to borrow some energy units from somewhere else in your life to apply to this work in the beginning. You may need to cut back some of your other activities for a while. Remember that you only have one hundred energy units to use every day. While you may not be thrilled about putting energy units into this work now, remember that later you will have extra energy units available every day because you won't be wasting them on the work of suppressing your emotions anymore.

Some people find that feeling their emotions is rather easy to do. Other people have done such an effective job of blocking their emotions that it can take months or even years for them to allow all their emotions to flow again. If you are a person who has trouble feeling your emotions, you will have to put more effort into this process.

Your objective is to learn what it feels like to feel your emotions again. What does your body feel like when you feel them? And how can you let them flow as easily as possible? To get things started, you can use exercises to trigger them. Try a number of different emotional triggers, and use the ones that feel right for you. Don't use the emotional triggers that don't resonate with you. Your goal isn't to start doing a bunch of rituals that don't have any meaning for you in the hope that eventually they will. If something isn't getting your emotions flowing, move on and try another trigger.

A number of things are effective for triggering emotions. Many emotional triggers are included here, and you may think of others as well. It would be good if you could find a few things that are especially effective triggers that you can depend on when you need to. In the beginning as you are relearning how to feel your emotions, you may find that sometimes you have trouble getting them flowing. You may feel unsettled and know you have something to feel, but you may be having trouble feeling it. If you have a trigger that you know is effective for you (for example, a sentimental music CD that always triggers sadness), you can use that on the days when it's tough to get your emotions flowing.

Movies and television shows are good triggers for emotions. You can watch a sad movie that makes you cry or a scary movie that makes you feel fear. You can watch a political talk show with a viewpoint that annoys you; instead of turning the channel, sit and watch that show and feel the anger it triggers. Try watching movies and television shows that you would typically avoid. You may find that you avoided them in the past because they triggered emotions you weren't comfortable with. Watch them now and feel those emotions.

Music is a good trigger for emotions. Listen to sappy love songs that make you cry. Listen to music that annoys you. For example, if you hate listening to loud rock music, sit still and listen to it and feel your anger. Listen to all different types of music, and find the types that affect you the most. Listen to songs from your past, and feel all the emotions in your emotional basement associated with those songs.

Looking at old pictures can trigger deep emotions. Photographs of a loved one who has died can trigger sadness. Pictures of someone who hurt you can trigger anger or fear. You will know that a person is connected to emotions in your emotional basement if pictures of them trigger intense emotions. Use their pictures as triggers to bring those emotions out.

Reading books can trigger emotions. Whether the stories are scary or funny or sad, they can trigger a lot of emotions. Listening to audiobooks may also be helpful because you can listen to the story without having to focus your mind on the words on the page. Fictional stories tend to be especially good at triggering emotions. Nonfiction can help too, as long as it isn't too factual or analytical. For example, maybe a biography or historical nonfiction book will bring out your emotions as you get involved in the drama of what has happened to the people in the story.

Breath work can help trigger emotions. People in our culture tend to breathe rapidly and shallowly. The process of taking some time out and paying attention to your breathing is a way of bringing yourself back into awareness of your body. Slowing down your breathing and consciously taking longer, deeper breaths is a simple way of calming your mind and triggering your emotions.

There are a number of breathing exercises you can do. You can simply close your eyes and slow down your breathing for a little while, or you can try more complicated breathing techniques. There are many books written about breath work. There are also meditation and yoga practices that work with the breath. If you find that you are interested in such techniques, investigate this area further until you find the ones that feel right for you. Remember that your goal with these exercises is to trigger emotions, not to focus your intellect on the details of the exercises.

As previously mentioned, you can use breath work to trigger anger. Instead of using slow deep breaths, you can do the rapid labor-style breathing to trigger anger. You can also use a swearword mantra. Repeat the mantra over and over again to get your anger flowing. As the anger flows, you can hit your pillow or shake your hands or do whatever safe actions are most helpful in keeping your anger flowing in a healthy way.

Dreams are good triggers for bringing out emotions. When you sleep at night, your intellect turns off and isn't as effective at holding the lid on your emotional organ closed. This allows you to feel your emotions more easily than you typically would during the day. If you wake up in the middle of the night from a nightmare and your heart is pounding, let yourself feel your fear. If you wake up from a sad dream or one that makes you angry, let yourself feel the sadness or the anger. If you have a joyful dream, let yourself feel the joy. The amount of emotion you will be able to feel in the middle of the night may depend on what time you have to wake up in the morning. You may not have hours to lie awake with your emotions flowing. You may have to feel them for just a little while and then go back to sleep. But you may find that if you don't let your emotions flow during the day, your body will insist on keeping you up at night to feel them.

Probably the most powerful triggers for our emotions are our dramas. Situations such as a fight with your spouse or a problem at work can trigger intense emotions. I'll talk about how to deal with your dramas in more depth later in this book. For now, start thinking about the bothersome situations in your life not only as problems to deal with but also as triggers for your emotions. For example, when someone says something to provoke your anger, it is tempting to try to figure out why she is doing what she is doing and how to change her. But with this new approach, you will want to start focusing inward on yourself instead.

When a person or situation triggers an emotion in you, you should temporarily put that person or situation in the background and feel the emotions that are triggered. Unless it is an emergency, don't do anything to fix the situation right away. Instead, step back and give yourself time to feel your emotions; you can take an action step to deal with the situation later. Start working to see everything in your life as, first and foremost, a lesson to help you understand yourself more deeply. A big part of this lesson is to feel the emotions that the situation triggers.

Sometimes you can't easily leave a situation that is triggering your emotions to go off by yourself to feel them. For example, your boss may make you angry or sad, but you can't just leave work and go home to feel your anger or sadness; you have to keep working. Staying in the situation will be easy to do once you've gotten the hang of feeling emotions. But maybe you haven't gotten comfortable enough yet with your emotions to both feel them and continue to function. Maybe you know that if you start to get angry you will want to huff and puff and swear up a storm. Or maybe if you are sad, you know you will start to cry your eyes out and you aren't comfortable doing that at work.

In such situations you can do one of two things. If you have the freedom to go somewhere to be alone, for example, a bathroom or some other private area, you can go there. You can spend a little time feeling your anger or sadness and decompressing your emotional organ a bit to make it easier to continue working. Later on, when you are at home you can remember the situation and feel your emotions more fully.

The second option, if it isn't possible for you to take time out to feel your emotions while you are at work, is to commit the details of the situation to your memory to refer back to later. Write them in a journal to remember them more clearly if you need to. For example, write down exactly what your boss said and did, and write down how you felt. When you get home from work and have time alone, you can remember the situation in as much detail as possible and try to retrigger the anger or sadness you weren't able to feel while you were at work.

With time you won't have to leave the situation to feel your emotions, but in the beginning you may need to do this. If you can't feel your emotions in a way that isn't dramatic and out of control, you shouldn't be feeling them in public. It can be easy to be judged or stigmatized when you feel your emotions in a dramatic way in public. And it can be easy to make messes that you will need to clean up later. You shouldn't put yourself at risk for all the stress that dramatic emotions cause. You also shouldn't make yourself vulnerable by feeling your emotions in front of people who don't understand what you are doing.

Another common trigger for emotions is illness. If you have a disease that causes you to have physical pain or other uncomfortable symptoms, you can use those symptoms as a trigger for your emotions. You can sit in silence with your symptoms and let yourself feel any sadness, anger, or fear that you have connected to them. If you are up in the middle of the night because of your pain, let yourself wallow in the pain. Let yourself cry, swear, or feel whatever is coming through you. Don't tell yourself to be strong. And don't tell yourself that everything will be all right. If you feel awful, let yourself feel awful. If you share a bed with someone, you may need to go into another room to allow yourself to feel your emotions without having to bother your bed partner.

Any time you are alone is a good time to trigger your emotions. When people are driving alone, they have time to reflect and focus on themselves. You may find that your time in the car is an ideal time to let your emotions flow. You can trigger them by listening to music or an audiobook. But be cautious if you find that your emotions are very intense. If they are so intense that you could become inattentive and have an accident, either pull over for a while or close the lid on your emotional organ until you can get out of the car.

It might be helpful for you to inform the people close to you that you are going to be using this new approach to feeling your emotions. Let them know that if they catch you crying or appearing angry, they don't need to worry about you. Explain that this is not about them or anything they are doing. Tell them that you will let them know when there is a problem you need to discuss with them, but for now everything is okay. This will hopefully take the pressure off you *and* them. You will be able to relax and feel your emotions without worrying about upsetting them, and they won't have to worry about why you have become more emotional.

While the process of feeling your emotions may feel unusual at first, over time you will get more comfortable with it. You will start to find that feeling emotions brings many welcome changes. You will feel more stable emotionally. You won't have to tighten up your muscles so much to hold the lid on your emotional organ closed, and this will help your physical pain and other uncomfortable symptoms. Feeling your emotions will also stimulate your energy flow.

The following exercises will help trigger your emotional flow. Try the ones that feel right for you.

▶*EXERCISE: Spend time watching movies and television shows to trigger your emotions. Laugh, cry, be angry, and be afraid. Watch movies you would usually avoid. If you usually avoid suspense films, make yourself watch something scary. If you usually avoid sad movies, make yourself watch something sappy. If you are uncomfortable feeling your emotions in front of other people, watch them by yourself.*

▶*EXERCISE: Go through your old music and listen to everything. Feel the emotions that are triggered. Also listen to the radio and try stations you normally wouldn't listen to. If hard rock with a pounding beat* usually annoys you, let yourself listen to that music and feel the anger it triggers. Borrow someone else's music or borrow music from the library to listen to a broader variety of sounds. Try opera and country and jazz and reggae. Hold on to the music that triggers your emotions the most, and listen to it when you need to.

▶EXERCISE: Read books that will trigger your emotions. Try romances, suspense novels, or whatever appeals to you. If you are going to use nonfiction, be careful; you don't want to waste your time getting too intellectual with this exercise. Read biographies and history books about people and situations that appeal to you emotionally.

▶EXERCISE: Go through your old photographs, scrapbooks, and memorabilia, and let yourself feel the emotions triggered by your memories.

▶EXERCISE: We tend to avoid situations that trigger emotions, so now think of situations you would normally avoid, and take part in them to trigger the emotions associated with them. For example, you may have grown up with a religion that you now avoid because you have much inner conflict over the beliefs you were taught. Now you could attend a religious service and feel the emotions it triggers for you. If you typically avoid reading the newspaper or watching news shows because the bad news in the world is upsetting, now you can read the newspaper or watch the news shows and use them as a trigger for your emotions. If there are television shows you avoid because they present a political view that is different than yours, watch those shows and feel the emotions they trigger.

Other examples would include going to a place that brings back a painful memory or calling a person who triggers emotions for you. You don't have to tell that person why you are calling or get into a drama with them. Just talk to them about superficial things to bring up the old memories and emotions.

▶*EXERCISE: Try some simple breathing exercises.*

1. Start by observing yourself. Sit or lie in a comfortable position, and pay attention to your breath, and just observe it. How fast are you breathing? Are you breathing deeply or more shallowly? What muscles do you use when you breathe?

2. Focus on breathing more slowly, more quietly, and more regularly. Allow your lungs to fill fully with air and then to deflate slowly like a balloon.

3. Try abdominal breathing: start your breath from your abdomen instead of your chest. Imagine a string attached to your belly button. As you inhale, let that string pull your abdomen out; this will pull your diaphragm down and open your lungs, allowing you to get a bigger breath of air. Slowly return your chest and abdomen back to normal as you exhale.

You may get dizzy or light-headed with these breathing exercises at first. If you do, stop and breathe regularly until the light-headedness is resolved.

You can do these exercises for relaxation for a few minutes, two or three times a day or whenever you feel stressed. You can use the breath work just to relax, but also to trigger emotions. If you are feeling that some emotion is trying to come through you but it is having trouble flowing, sit or lie quietly and breathe. You may be able to use your breath work to bring out the emotion. Once the emotion is triggered, allow it to flow through your body.

▶*EXERCISE: Do a more rapid labor-style breathing—whoo-whoo, whoo-whoo—to trigger your anger (slow down your breath if you get light-headed). Find a swearword or another acceptable word or phrase to be your anger mantra; sit by yourself and repeat the mantra to help bring your anger out. You can also shake your hands, hit your bed with a sock roll, or punch a pillow. But remember: never hurt yourself or others when you are feeling anger.*

Another thing you can do to trigger anger is to write a word, such as mad, *over and over on a piece of paper. Or just scribble; the process of scribbling can help you bypass your intellect and let your emotions flow.*

▶ EXERCISE: *It is common to feel unsettled emotionally and not know what you are feeling. When you are in a situation that makes you emotionally uneasy, ask yourself what a child would feel in this situation. A child wouldn't stop to think about why he feels an emotion. He would just go ahead and feel it. By imagining what a child would feel, you may be able to identify what you are feeling.*

▶ EXERCISE: *Use your dreams at night as a trigger for your emotions. If you aren't letting your emotions flow during the day, they may come out at night when you wake up from a dream. Don't try to calm yourself when you wake up from a scary or sad dream; instead, let your emotions flow.*

▶ EXERCISE: *As you work with emotional triggers, keep a list of the ones that work best. When you are in pain, having insomnia, or having other physical symptoms, consult your list and use the trigger that will best help you get your emotions flowing. It is healthier to feel your emotions in these situations than to sit quietly and suffer physically.*

▶ EXERCISE: *Remember that one of the most powerful triggers of emotions is our dramas. When a situation or another person triggers an emotion in you, step back from the situation and focus on feeling the emotion. Unless you have an urgent situation that needs immediate action, leave the action step for later and feel your emotions instead.*

Special Issues with Emotions
Although feeling emotions in this new way is not dangerous, if you have a history of severe physical or emotional trauma, you may need support from your family and your medical providers as you start to work on letting your emotions flow. It is common for people to

tightly close the lid on the emotional organ after trauma, and this causes emotions to become pent up inside you. As you open the lid on the emotional organ, your body can be so relieved to release your emotions that it may be a bit shocking for you at first, especially if you have had your emotions closed tightly in the emotional basement for a long time. Your mind may have trouble accepting your emotional flow, and your body may be uncomfortable in the beginning as it is learning how to feel emotions again. You may initially have a sense of being out of control, and this may take some time to get used to. You may want to have someone with you when you are feeling overwhelmed by the emotions. Over time you will get more comfortable with what your body is doing, and it won't feel so foreign to you anymore.

If you have a history of dramatic actions, such as suicide attempts or other self-injurious behaviors, you will need to make sure that you don't hurt yourself as you work on feeling your emotions in this new way. Remember that it is never healthy to hurt yourself or anyone else when you are feeling your emotions. People can turn on themselves and harm themselves because they don't know how to let their emotions flow in a healthy way. You may need support as you learn how to let your emotions flow without hurting yourself.

Having a psychiatric illness is not a reason to avoid feeling your emotions. Blocked emotions are actually a cause of some psychiatric disorders, and feeling your emotions will help heal those disorders. Anxiety is an example of a psychiatric illness caused in part by suppressed emotions. Many people get into the habit of suppressing their fear. They hold it in until it builds up and floods out and causes intense physical symptoms, such as hyperventilation and chest pain. This intense emotional flow commonly gets labeled as anxiety. As people with anxiety start to feel their fear in a healthy way and let it flow on a regular basis, their intense physical symptoms of anxiety improve. Another cause of anxiety is a hyperactive intellect. I'll discuss that in the next chapter.

Depression is another psychiatric illness that is frequently caused by the suppression of healthy emotional flow. Actually depression can be considered an emotion too. People who are depressed feel it physically in their bodies the way they feel the other emotions. But depression is different from other emotions because, while it is healthy to feel the other emotions as much as is needed, it is not regenerative or healthy to be chronically depressed. People who are chronically depressed live in a gray, empty world that is not energetically balanced, so staying in a state of depression is not healthy.

Depression may be caused by genetics or an imbalance in brain chemistry. It can also be caused by the suppression of healthy emotional flow. If you don't let your sadness, anger, fear, and joy flow in a spontaneous, unobstructed way, you will develop an imbalance in your energy flow and start to get fatigued and depressed. While you may need to take antidepressants to control your depression, by feeling your healthy emotions you may be able to get to the root of the problem and heal it.

Another common cause of depression is an unhealthy life situation. While you are feeling your emotions, you also need to work on identifying and healing life situations that are out of balance for you. Feeling your emotions won't be enough to cure your depression if you feel trapped in an impossible relationship or a bad job. In those cases you will need to feel your emotions *and* change the situation.

As you start to work on feeling your emotions, be aware that many drugs block emotional flow or change the way you experience your emotions. These drugs include alcohol, recreational drugs, and a number of prescription medications. People using these substances may think they are feeling their emotions, but the emotional flow isn't a healthy, healing experience. While people are using these substances, their emotional flow can be blocked and they may try to feel their emotions but they can't. Or these substances can change the way that they feel their emotions, and they may get confused and think that they are feeling healthy emotions when their emotions aren't actually flowing in a healthy way. Or these substances can cause people to lose control of their actions and project their emotions and become violent.

Alcohol and recreational drugs can be very problematic when you are trying to feel your emotions in a healthy way. To feel your emotions most effectively, you should stop using them. If you have trouble stopping them on your own, you should get advice from your physician on how to stop them or safely taper off them. Be aware that if you regularly drink large amounts of alcohol, the withdrawal syndrome can be dangerous and possibly life threatening, so you should get assistance as you consider stopping it. You may need to go through chemical-dependency treatment for support when you are stopping alcohol and recreational drugs.

A number of prescription medications can be unhealthy because of the way they affect emotional flow. Pain medications in the opioid family (for example, morphine, Oxycontin, methadone, and hydrocodone) blunt emotional flow. While these medications are very effective at treating pain, especially when used for short periods of time, they can be detrimental when used over long periods of time. In addition to other side effects, their tendency to block emotions limits the ability of patients taking them to actively work on their healing.

Other prescription medications, such as antidepressants (for example, Prozac, Zoloft, Celexa, and Effexor) and benzodiazepines (for example, Valium, Ativan, and Klonopin), also blunt emotional flow. The purpose of these drugs is to bring brain chemistry back into balance in patients with psychiatric diseases, including depression and anxiety. There are situations in which these medications are necessary, especially in patients with severe psychiatric symptoms. But because these drugs have a tendency to block emotions, in the long run they can inhibit your ability to heal.

If you are on prescription drugs and you find that they are inhibiting your emotional flow, you should discuss tapering off them with your physician. Many of these drugs have uncomfortable withdrawal syndromes, and some can also have life-threatening withdrawal syndromes, so don't just stop them on your own. As you taper off them, you will find that your emotions will start to flow more easily. If you find that you can't taper off the addictive prescription drugs, you may need chemical-dependency treatment.

While the process of feeling emotions is a healthy, natural one, it can be difficult in the beginning. It can be uncomfortable to deal with the physical sensations that come with feeling your emotions at first, and your mind can have a hard time accepting that it is healthy to feel them. You may have had past experiences that have affected your understanding of your emotions. You may have trouble embracing the idea of opening the lid on the emotional organ and cleaning out your emotional basement. No matter what issues make you tentative about the idea of feeling emotions, remember that healthy emotional flow is vital for healthy energy flow, physical health, and inner peace.

4   The Intellect

The intellect is another aspect of your inner self that needs to be brought into balance for you to have healthy energy flow. The intellect is the computerlike part of your mind that deals with language, logic, and complex thinking tasks. It performs the thought processes that help you function. You use your intellect when you talk, read, and write. It guides you when you are performing tasks, such as bathing, dressing, and preparing meals. It helps you figure out how to drive your car or run your computer.

Without your intellect, you wouldn't be able to solve complicated problems. You wouldn't be able to figure out how to balance your budget, learn foreign languages, or do your job. Your intellect helps with the thinking tasks that you do every day.

The intellect is the part of you that thinks all your thoughts. If you are sitting in a meeting or a class and you are bored, your intellect is the part of you that starts thinking about other things, such as what you're going to eat for dinner or when you're going to do your laundry. Your intellect looks back into the past to remember the movie you watched last night. It imagines what you could be doing right now instead of what you're actually doing.

Your intellect is the part of you that has an imagination and tells stories. It looks at the world around you and analyzes what it sees. It tries to make sense of the experiences you have. For example, if your house burns down, your intellect will try to figure out why this happened. It might not always know the whole answer, but it will try to figure things out as clearly as it can with the information it is given.

Your intellect makes you aware that you are an individual and different from the people around you. Another word for this aspect of the intellect is *ego*. It compares you to the people around you and tells you how you add up. It makes judgments about whether you are better than other people or inadequate compared to them. It tells you how you should think and act in order to fit in.

Our intellects do amazing things, and we have used them to change our world. But they also have some unhealthy habits that are harmful for us. These habits bring our energy flow out of balance. You will need to identify your intellect's unhealthy habits and work to calm them to bring your energy flow back into healthy balance.

One troublesome habit the intellect has is the habit of thinking too much. Of course we want our intellects to do their work to figure things out. If we have bills to pay, we want our intellects to figure out how much to pay and how to write the checks. But once that is done, our intellects should be able to stop and take a break. Unfortunately, once the intellect starts thinking, it can be hard for it to stop and rest.

Imagine your intellect inside your head chattering incessantly, as though it's running on a thought treadmill. There often seems to be a powerful magnet holding the intellect in place on the treadmill. It continues to run nonstop, unable to slow down, unable to get off. You may be lying in bed at night trying to fall sleep, and one thought after another will come randomly into your head. No matter how hard you tell yourself to stop thinking, you just can't. You might be thinking, *Did I handle the assignment from my boss the right way? Did I make productive comments at the meeting today, or did I sound stupid? Can anyone tell that I've gained weight? Did I remember to close the garage door?*

When you are on the thought treadmill, your intellect may shift from one topic to another or obsess about one specific subject.

THE INTELLECT

Whatever you are thinking about can seem so important that you can have trouble breaking yourself free from that thought. You may find yourself spending hours on end thinking and thinking and thinking. At times it can seem impossible to get off the intellectual treadmill.

When your intellect is running on the thought treadmill, it can affect your physical body. You can develop insomnia because your intellect can't turn off at night. It is also common for people to tighten up their muscles when their intellects are in overdrive. This can lead to muscle pain. Some people clench their jaws and get jaw pain and headaches. Some people tighten their neck or back muscles and get pain in their necks and backs. Some people tighten the muscles in their pelvises and rectums and get pain in those areas.

Some people have anxiety caused by intellectual hyperactivity. Sometimes anxiety is caused by suppressed fear, but anxiety can also be triggered by a hyperactive intellect. If you have persistent thoughts and your intellect can't get off the thought treadmill, you can become almost paralyzed and have trouble functioning. If you have anxiety, you should identify what exactly your anxiety consists of: physical fear, intellectual hyperactivity, or both. You can apply the information from the chapter on emotions to learn how to feel your physical fear in a healthier way. The information in this chapter will help you work on calming your intellectual hyperactivity.

Western culture, in particular, focuses on the intellect. We are always trying to figure things out. We are constantly searching for more information. We always want evidence to back up our beliefs. We continually push our intellects to work harder and harder. Unfortunately, the more we push our intellects to work, the harder it gets for us to allow them to stop and rest. And as our intellects get busier, they push our bodies to work harder too.

To be healthy, you need to have a healthy balance between activity and rest. This applies to your physical body and to your intellect. If you don't let your body stop and rest, it will wear out. If you don't let your intellect stop and rest, it will cause you to lose your inner peace. This is a hard concept for our culture to appreciate. We have a tendency to live on the treadmill, physically and intellectually.

To truly rest, you need to be able to rest your body *and* your intellect. Resting your intellect while continuing to work your body into exhaustion isn't healthy. And resting your body while running your intellect on the intellectual treadmill isn't healthy either. Only when you can rest both can you find a healthy balance in your life.

An important aspect of the relationship between your intellect and your body is the mind-body connection. New Age proponents talk a lot about the mind-body connection. At times this concept can seem too mystical and otherworldly for the average person to appreciate, but there is a very simple nuts-and-bolts approach you can take toward your mind-body connection that can be very helpful.

Imagine that your body is like your car. Just as your car moves you around from one place to another, your body moves your consciousness around from one place to another. The big difference between your body and your car is that you can get out of your car and exchange it for a new one. But your consciousness is stuck in your body until you die, and you can't trade it in. Even if you are a quadriplegic and can't move around, your body is still the vehicle that you are sitting in while you are on this earth.

Your car needs fuel and maintenance work. The fuel for your car is gasoline; the maintenance work includes things such as oil changes and tire rotations. If you don't do those things, your car won't run well. You will also need to do extra work if your car breaks down. If you don't fix it, you will be stuck at home and won't be able to go anywhere.

Your body is more sophisticated than your car, but it works the same basic way. Its fuel requirements include things such as energy, air, food, and water. It needs maintenance in the form of exercise and rest. Each of our bodies has its own specific requirements to keep it healthy. Different bodies have different diet, exercise, and rest requirements. Some bodies may like to run marathons, whereas others prefer to walk or swim. Some bodies need seven hours of sleep, whereas others need nine.

Imagine yourself sitting behind the steering wheel of your car. You decide where your car will go and how you will get there. In a similar way, your intellect sits inside your brain and drives your body. It tells your body where to go and when to go there. It tells your body when to sleep and when to wake up. It decides what kind of fuel your body will take in and how that fuel will be spent. It decides whether your body will take up skydiving or take a trip to China. When you think of the phrase *mind-body connection,* think of the mind as the intellect making the executive decisions and the body as the car that follows the orders the intellect gives.

The problem for both your car and your body comes when you don't take good care of them. It can be easy to be an irresponsible owner and neglect your car and forget to change the oil. Or you may drive too fast on bumpy roads and break an axle. The same thing happens with your body. Your intellect doesn't always care about what your body needs. It has a tendency to make decisions without listening to your body's input. It decides that what it wants is more important. It may decide that it doesn't have time to cook healthy meals, so it makes your body eat food that is easy to prepare but that upsets your stomach. It may decide that it has too much to do, so it makes your body get only six hours of sleep when it really needs nine. Sooner or later your body is going to pay the price of your intellect's expectations by getting fatigued or sick.

The relationship between your mind and your body is like any other relationship. There can be a conflict when one of the members of the relationship neglects or abuses the other. When your intellect neglects your body, you can refer to it as your *mind-body conflict.* A good example of the mind-body conflict can be observed in some people who run marathons. Many runners are experienced and prepare for marathons in a healthy way. The conflict comes for the people who aren't regular runners and who just wake up one day and say that they're going to run a marathon. Their intellects may decide that it will sound really good if they can say they ran a marathon. And maybe they think that will prove how tough and athletic they are. But if they don't have bodies that tolerate running long distances or if they are in poor condition, there will be a problem. They are setting themselves up for a huge mind-body conflict.

Our bodies try their best to do what our intellects tell them to do. They are like dogs that want to please their caretakers. So on the day of the marathon, even if you aren't really up to the challenge, your body does its best to finish the race. The experience may be grueling and miserable. Your body may develop injuries and may feel like stopping at mile seventeen, but your intellect keeps pushing it forward so it can say that you crossed the finish line. By the last mile, your body may be dehydrated and need intravenous fluids and you may hardly be able to walk, but your intellect keeps driving your body forward. For two weeks following the marathon, your body may be in pain and you may be walking with a limp, but your intellect is so thrilled that it can brag "I finished that marathon!" that it overlooks the fact that it abused your body.

Your intellect gets a lot of ideas regarding what it wants your body to do. Sometimes those ideas are good for both your intellect and your body, but often they put your body in a place of imbalance. The important thing to understand about your body is that it wants to please your intellect. It is programmed to follow orders from the driver the same way your car is. The body can take a lot of abuse, but it can only take so much abuse before it eventually breaks down.

We've all had times when our intellects had plans or expectations that our bodies couldn't meet. If your intellect continually ignores your body's needs because it thinks that its own are more important, you will eventually develop an imbalance in your energy flow. This will lead to illness. Each individual body has its own threshold for how much neglect and abuse it can take before it starts to break down. Some people have physical constitutions that allow them to work heavy-labor jobs for decades before they start to deteriorate, but eventually they start to pay the price. Other people's bodies are more sensitive and tolerate much less stress before they start to get sick and wear out. They may start to have pain and other illnesses early in their lives.

Our culture reinforces the idea that our minds should abuse our bodies. We are taught to always push ourselves to the limit and push beyond our pain and exhaustion. Of course there are times when you have to push your body beyond what is healthy, but you should limit those times as much as possible. Unfortunately, people have a tendency to continue to push themselves even when it is possible for them to slow down and find more balance.

If you observe the changes in our culture over the last century, you will be able to easily understand why people are having such a difficult time bringing their mind-body conflict to an end. For tens of thousands of years, people had to work hard physically to survive. They had to grow or hunt their own food. They had to work hard to find sources of energy to heat their homes. They had to do all their work without the advantage of modern machines. They didn't have indoor plumbing, electricity, or any of the modern conveniences we take for granted. Because people lived that way for so many centuries, they got into the habit of expecting to work hard physically. They got used to pushing their bodies to get things done; they knew they wouldn't survive if they didn't push to keep going.

Over the last century, our intellects have helped us make great strides with advances in many areas, including industry and technology. We have created machines to help us do almost everything. We can use machines to harvest crops rather than having to do it by hand. We have cars that get us places in a fraction of the time it would take with a horse and buggy. We have machines that make almost everything easier and faster. These new machines have given us the luxury of extra time and energy to spend on things other than the struggle to put food on our tables and shelters over our heads.

One would think that with the amazing advances we've made in the last century, we'd all be relaxing and enjoying life a little bit more. Unfortunately, the very intellects that helped us improve our world are now hurting us. In an ideal world, our intellects would realize that we can relax now and enjoy our lives. Instead, they are having trouble letting go of the old messages that tell us to push ourselves and abuse our bodies. They just don't seem to realize yet that we can relax and survive more easily than we did when we had to do things the hard way.

One way our intellects have found to keep pushing us is to create new messages about the things we must do. Our intellects tell us that we should work long hours so we can afford big houses and fancy cars. They tell us we need to compete with other people to be richer, smarter, stronger, faster, or more successful than they are. There are countless stories floating around in our culture telling us how we should be and what we should do. We wouldn't necessarily need to believe these stories, but we get in the habit of believing them. Most of these stories don't involve a life-or-death survival situation, like finding our next meal, but our intellects trick us into thinking that they do.

As you are working on healing yourself, you will need to calm your intellect. You will need to identify and let go of the stories that tell you to push yourself to do things that are unhealthy for you. You will need to learn to step off the intellectual treadmill and let your intellect take a rest. You will also need to resolve your mind-body conflicts. Only when you calm your intellect will you be able to bring your energy flow back into healthy balance.

▶*EXERCISE: Notice how busy you are. Can you sit quietly for thirty minutes without the television or computer on or without doing anything specific? Do you ever just stop and let your mind and your body rest? Can you hang out in your house all day or all weekend in your pajamas and not accomplish anything important? You can use this exercise as a diagnostic test to teach you about yourself. If you can't stop and rest and simply waste some time, you can assume that your intellect is probably* overly active. If you find that you don't ever give yourself a chance to rest, start scheduling time to do it.

▶ EXERCISE: Try taking a break from using your cell phone, computer, television, and electronic devices for a few hours or a few days. You can assume that you have an overly active intellect if you can't spend time without them. If you find that you have trouble spending time without them, take short breaks at first and extend them as tolerated. You don't have to stop watching television or using your computer, but if these devices are running your life, you need to bring the situation into healthier balance.

▶ EXERCISE: How good of a listener are you? When people are poor listeners it is often because they are too busy thinking to listen. For one day, consciously observe how easy it is for you to listen to what other people are saying without interrupting them. If you notice yourself interrupting others a lot, your intellect may be in overdrive.

▶ EXERCISE: Pay attention to your sleep. If you have trouble falling asleep at night, your intellect may be too hyperactive during the day to allow you to relax and fall asleep at night. Another part of the problem may be that your intellect is driving your body to be too busy during the day, and your body can have a hard time relaxing at night as well. Give yourself time in the evening to relax your intellect and body before bed.

▶ EXERCISE: Take a long look at your body in the mirror, and recognize it for what it is: the vehicle that is transporting you through your life. Let yourself really focus on the state of your body, and hear what it is saying to you. Does it need a change? Does it have symptoms that are trying to warn you that you need to change your priorities? This exercise isn't about judging what your body looks like. Instead, your focus should be about your need to honor and respect your body for the life it gives you.

▶EXERCISE: Start watching the way your intellect and your body interact. Do you find yourself pushing your body to do things it doesn't want to do? Does your body complain with fatigue or pain or other symptoms when you push it too hard? Do you wake up in the morning feeling awful, and do you need to start dosing yourself with coffee or medications to force yourself through your day? When your body complains, does your intellect tell it to shut up and keep going?

▶EXERCISE: Listen to the stories you tell yourself as you try to justify the things you do to neglect your body. For example, is your job or a relationship or a hobby more important than your body's needs? You may not be ready to change anything big overnight, but start paying attention, and find little ways you can be more caring toward your body. Can you skip some housework and go to bed an hour earlier? Can you change your work schedule and go for a walk before work? Even if you don't have enough energy to follow through with the changes yet, start watching for potential changes you could make.

The Balance Between the Intellect and the Emotions

A vital part of the relationship between the intellect and the body is the relationship between the intellect and the emotions. Remember that the intellect is the computerlike part of your mind that thinks and analyzes and tells stories. Your emotions are physical, in your body. People commonly confuse the intellect for emotions. They think that talking about emotions and analyzing them counts as feeling them, but it doesn't. Emotions are experienced physically, and they don't need any words to describe them at all.

While the intellect can tell stories and analyze the world, it isn't able to truly experience the world on a physical level. It needs our bodies and our emotions to do that. Think about the difference between playing a hockey game on a computer and playing the game in real life. The intellect is the part of you that would play the game on the computer. When you are playing on the computer, you can see your player

THE INTELLECT

moving the puck around on the screen and you can tell stories about the game, but you can't physically feel the weight of the hockey stick in your hands. On the other hand, your body is the part of you that would play the game in real life. When you are playing on a real rink, you feel the physical sensation of skating, the ice sliding beneath your skates, and the stick maneuvering the puck. You have a much richer physical experience playing the game in real life compared to playing on the computer because your entire body is involved.

For optimal health we need both our intellects and our physical bodies to function in a healthy way. It is important that we use our intellects to analyze and solve problems, and we also need to let our emotions flow in a healthy way. We need to have both of these parts of our inner selves in balance to be healthy. Unfortunately, it is common for people to allow their intellects to become too active. Their intellects then have a tendency to choke off their emotional flow and bring the system out of balance.

Imagine a balance for measuring weights, its two arms at the top extending outward from the center and a tray hanging from each arm. Picture the emotions on one tray and the intellect on the other. The two trays need to be in balance for us to have healthy energy flow. Most people have an imbalance; the intellect side of the balance is excessively weighed down with hyperactive thoughts, and the emotion side of the balance is weightless, dangling up in the air because of blocked emotional flow.

The intellect brings the system out of balance by judging emotions as bad and stopping emotional flow. Recall the image of the emotional organ with the lid on top. The intellect sits in your head above the emotional organ and uses its intellectual messages to hold the lid closed so your emotions can't get out. When your intellect uses harmful messages, such as *Fear and anger are dangerous; don't feel them or you will get in trouble,* you tighten up your muscles and do whatever you need to do to keep the lid closed and stop your emotional flow.

In the beginning when you start to tell yourself that you want to fully feel your emotions again, you may feel a sense of stress and inner conflict. This is because once your body starts to feel the relief of letting your emotions flow, it will fight to allow the lid on your emotional organ to stay open. At the same time, your intellect may have trouble letting go of its bully position. It will fight to maintain control and try to keep the lid on your emotional organ tightly closed. This fight between your emotions and your intellect can make you feel very physically and emotionally uncomfortable.

It can be hard at first to bring your intellectual activity and your emotional flow into balance. The dynamics between these two parts of your inner self have been in place since you were a child, so it may take some time to change them. But you will find that if you recognize this interaction and work at calming your unhealthy intellectual messages, your intellect will start to realize that it can peacefully coexist with your emotions. With time it will get easier for your intellect to take a break and rest.

In our culture, the imbalance between the intellect and the emotions starts when we are young. When we are small, we are little bundles of emotions and energy. Our neurological systems are still immature and our intellectual activity is very limited. We are more focused on what we are feeling than what we are thinking. When a baby is hungry, he doesn't have the ability to analyze the situation and figure out how to fix a bottle. He just cries because his stomach is empty. When he is happy, he doesn't have the intellectual capacity to analyze why he is happy. He just laughs. Young children live in a state of spontaneous emotional flow with high energy flow.

As children grow older, their intellects become more developed. As the neuronal connections in their brains and bodies become stronger, they learn how to walk and talk. They get toilet trained and learn how to feed and dress themselves. They learn all the functions that they need to live and thrive.

As children's intellects develop, they become sponges, taking in and processing information from their environment. They copy the words and behaviors of the adults around them. They learn how to identify everything and give it a name. They learn that their toes are called *toes* and that their nose is called a *nose*. They learn that the process of moving around upright on two feet with one foot moving in front of the other is called *walking* and that saying words out loud is called *talking*.

They intuitively know that to survive, they need to fit in with the people around them. They use cues from those people to help them figure out what to do. They learn to say *please* and *thank you* and to follow other rules of etiquette. They learn that pulling their sister's hair is wrong. They learn not to steal other children's toys. As they grow up, they get thousands of messages from their parents, teachers, friends, television, and everyone they come in contact with. These messages tell them how they should think, feel, talk, and act in order to fit in.

One of the important things children get taught as their intellects are developing is how to suppress their emotions. Adults are uncomfortable with emotions because they haven't learned how to feel them in a healthy way themselves, so they continually tell their children that emotions are bad and unhealthy. Children start to believe the message that emotions are bad because they need approval from adults to fit in. They hear such messages as *Crying is for babies, so stop whining* or *Everything is okay, don't be sad* or *Big kids aren't scared* or *Don't get mad at your brother*. Although it is healthy to feel emotions, because their parents are uncomfortable with emotions, children learn to suppress emotions too.

It may be hard at first for children to believe the judgment that emotions are bad, but when they continually hear it, they start to believe it's true. They also may get punished if they can't control their emotions, and this reinforces the message. Over time they don't need adults to tell them to stop feeling their emotions; they learn to suppress them on their own. They analyze themselves and remember the message that they're bad if they cry or are angry, and their intellects override the emotions and send them to be stored down in the emotional basement. Over time their intellects get more weight and their emotions become more suppressed, and this is how the imbalance between the two develops.

▶*EXERCISE: Start observing the two different parts of your inner self: your emotions and your intellect. See how your emotions are physical and how your intellect does your thinking. Pay attention to the differences between the two. Recognize your emotional organ functioning when you are feeling something, and recognize your intellect as it thinks your thoughts.*

We often consider our intellectual messages to be emotions when they are really thoughts. For example, you may think, I feel so criticized by my mother. That is the intellectual message, but the emotion is the sadness or anger that you physically feel in reaction to your mother's criticism. Identify the difference between your emotions and your intellect as you go through your day.

▶*EXERCISE: Imagine your emotional organ with the lid on top. See how your intellect has a habit of holding the lid closed. Imagine your intellect relaxing its hold on the lid of your emotional organ and see your emotions being allowed to flow in a healthy way.*

▶*EXERCISE: Visualize a balance with its two trays, and picture your emotions on one tray and your intellect on the other. How is the balance between the two?*

▶*EXERCISE: Think back to when you were a child, and identify unhealthy intellectual messages you were taught about feeling emotions. Remember situations where you let yourself feel your emotions, and remember other situations where you learned to suppress them. Try not to judge the adults who taught you those messages. Remember that they didn't understand the whole dynamic between the intellect and the* emotions. *They were probably teaching you what they had been taught. Understanding where these unhealthy messages came from can help you let them go.*

Tribal Messages
Our culture teaches us all types of intellectual messages, not just unhealthy judgments about emotion. These messages serve many purposes. Some of them help us learn how to do all the things we need to do to take care of ourselves. We learn how to bathe and dress ourselves, and we learn how to take care of our homes and our possessions. Parents teach children messages such as *Wash behind your ears* and *You should floss your teeth every day*. Some intellectual messages are created for our safety, for example, *Don't swallow poison* and *Don't play with matches*. Some of them are created to help us know how to get along with other people, for example, *Hitting your friends is a bad thing to do*.

Other intellectual messages have been developed to help us fit into our tribes. Humans are tribal animals. Our tribes are vitally important to us all. When we are born, we need our tribes to take care of us and to help us survive. And we spend our lives in our tribes, socializing and sharing responsibilities with each other.

We are all members of tribes, whether we realize it or not. Our tribes include all the groups of people we associate with. Most of us belong to a number of different tribes. We belong to our family tribes and our local, regional, and national community tribes. We belong to our hometown tribe, our state tribe, and the United States tribe. With the recent trend toward globalization, our world is becoming a global community in which all humans belong to the earth tribe.

The people we work with are part of our work tribes. We also belong to tribes made up of our groups of friends. Whenever a group of people spends time together and shares a common purpose, those people experience a tribal association with each other. A group of vegetarians who all go to the same grocery store and talk together about their vegetarian beliefs is a vegetarian tribe. A group of quilters who get together regularly and sew is a quilting tribe.

The people in some of the tribes you belong to will spend time together. They will see each other at church or at baseball games. Their members will know each other personally, and they will do specific activities together and socialize with each other. The members of other tribes you belong to may not socialize with each other. They may not even live in the same geographical area. They belong to the same tribe because of their shared beliefs or other shared characteristics. Groups of people with similar religious and political beliefs belong to the tribes that share their beliefs. People who believe in the Catholic doctrine belong to the Catholic tribe, and people who believe in the Muslim doctrine belong to the Muslim tribe. People who agree with Democratic Party's political beliefs belong to the Democratic tribe, and people who agree with the Republican Party's political beliefs belong to the Republican tribe.

Everyone belongs to specific racial and ethnic tribes. Whites belong to the white tribe, and blacks belong to the black tribe. Within those tribes are a number of specific ethnic tribes, depending on where in the world your ancestors came from. You may belong to the American Italian tribe or the Ashkenazi Jewish tribe. Some people have strong associations with their racial and ethnic tribes, whereas other people feel that these tribal associations are not as important to them.

People of a similar social class or educational level belong to the same tribes. Rich people belong to the rich tribe, and poor people belong to the poor tribe. In the United States, there is also a middle-class tribe between the rich and the poor. People who have graduated from college belong to the college-graduate tribe. People in the military belong to their specific military-branch tribes.

People also belong to tribes that share their beliefs. For example, antiabortionists belong to the tribe that believes abortion is wrong. People who don't believe in global warming belong to the global-warming-is-a-lie tribe.

THE INTELLECT

It doesn't matter why you become part of your tribes. It doesn't matter if it is because you are born into them or if you choose to join them because you share a specific interest, belief, or purpose with them. The important thing to recognize is how deeply your tribes affect you. You can feel a great sense of security when you are part of a tribe. If you are part of a labor union and your employer threatens to fire you, you can depend on the union tribe to stand by you and protect you. If you are a child in school who is scared of being bullied by another child, you may ask your best friend to hang out with you at recess so you can feel the protection of your tribe of friends. There is a sense that because you share something with the other members in your tribe, you have their support and protection.

Another thing that people get from their tribes is a guide to how they should look, think, and act. It can be a relief to not have to be your own expert. Instead, you can ask your tribe to be your expert. If you are in high school and a new kid joins your class, you don't have to decide for yourself if you are going to be friends with the new kid. You can just wait and see how your tribe of friends treats the new kid and follow their lead.

Your tribes use intellectual messages to tell you everything about how you should live, from how much money you should make to what kind of house you should buy to how many children you should have. They tell you how to dress and how to wear your hair. They tell you what you should eat and drink. They tell you how many hours you should work and how you should spend your free time. It can be a relief to let your tribes tell you what to do when you have a decision to make.

Although your tribes can give you a sense of security and belonging, there is also a dark side to belonging to tribes, and that is that they tend to require everyone to take a one-size-fits-all approach to life. If a tribe's beliefs are important to it, everyone in the tribe needs to agree with those beliefs. If the tribe values a certain appearance, you need to look like everyone else in the tribe to belong. If the tribe has a certain activity that is important to it, you need to do that activity to fit in.

Fitting into your tribe is fine if what they tell you to think and do is healthy and regenerative for you as an individual. But needing to fit in becomes a problem if your tribe's beliefs and actions aren't supportive of you. You can't find inner peace or physical health if you are following a tribe whose agenda doesn't support you as an individual.

The importance of the intellectual messages we learn from our tribes cannot be overestimated. Every aspect of our lives is affected by these messages. We learn thousands of them during our lifetimes. We are constantly thinking thoughts based on these messages. They are major motivating factors for our words and our actions.

While there are many healthy intellectual messages we learn from our tribes, they teach us many harmful ones too. One example of a harmful intellectual message tribes commonly teach their members is that you, as an individual, are not capable of being your own expert. Tribes teach their members that they don't have the insight or intelligence to make decisions for themselves. Members are taught that they have to let the tribe be their expert. This makes sense, because if tribes allow their members to be their own experts, their members may start questioning what the tribes are telling them. Their members may try to change the tribes if they don't like what the tribes tell them to say and do. Or they may decide to leave the tribes, and tribes don't want to lose members.

Other harmful intellectual messages people learn from their tribes are *I am not good enough* or *I am not acceptable the way that I am* or *There is something wrong with me*. Frequently people get taught these messages when they aren't fitting in well with their tribes. For example, you may be the one child in your family who doesn't do as well in sports or with grades as your siblings do. Or you may have less money than other people in your tribe and you can't afford to buy the expensive things they can. When you don't look or act as the other members in your tribe do, they may teach you that there is something wrong with you. As with the message telling people that they can't be their own experts, tribes use these critical messages to keep their members in place. They want to keep you feeling inadequate so you won't make trouble and won't have the confidence to leave and find a tribe you are more comfortable with.

When tribes are teaching messages to make their members feel inadequate, sometimes they do it in a very obvious way. They may say out loud, "You are a failure." But often these messages are much more subtle. The other members of your tribe may not say anything specific, but their actions will let you know that you are different and inadequate. They may give you a critical look or ignore you when you are asking them for help. These subtle messages can be more difficult to identify than the obvious insults, but they can be just as harmful. Over time they can slowly erode a tribal member's sense of self-confidence. This starts a cycle in which the member feels less and less confident and less and less able to leave the tribe, even when he or she is being hurt by the tribe.

People get in the habit of thinking that they can't survive without their tribes. It makes sense that people would think this. Until recently people really were dependent on their tribes for survival. They needed to pool their resources and work together every day to find food and shelter and to take care of all their basic needs. If they didn't get the crops in or if they didn't get shelters built before winter, they could die. They realized that they had to work together and allow their tribes to make the rules about how they should live to make things work more successfully.

But as Western culture has evolved over the last century, we've gained the ability for individuals to have more independence. We can go to the grocery store to buy our food and other necessities. With the global economy, we have a seemingly unlimited number of choices regarding what we can buy at the store. We don't need to depend on our tribes to help us do everything as we did in the past.

We also have many options regarding what type of work we can do now. In the past, men were typically forced to follow career paths their families chose for them and women were limited to being housewives, teachers, or nurses. Now men *and* women can choose for themselves the careers that are most satisfying for them. All the lifestyle options currently available to us give us an incredible number of choices. We don't have to stay in tribes that are unhealthy for us, and we don't have to believe intellectual messages that aren't healthy for us.

Although we currently have the potential to leave unhealthy tribes and let go of unhealthy tribal messages, it is a very hard thing to do. It is hard to break free from our tribes, even if they are hurting us. It's almost as if humans have been dependent on their tribes for so long that this dependence has become part of the human body and our cellular memory. Deep inside us are still the people who know winter is coming, the crop isn't in yet, and there is not enough firewood, so they'd better hold on to their tribe for a little while longer to be safe. Even if our tribes hurt us, we still think, deep down, that maybe the alternative is worse. So we hold on to our tribes and the messages they teach us, even when those messages are unhealthy.

As tribes evolve, so do the intellectual messages their members believe in. For example, in the past (and in many cultures still today) there were well-defined expectations regarding the roles of men and women in society. Intellectual messages such as *Men are the head of the household* and *Women should always defer to their husbands' judgment* were commonly accepted. As the relationship between men and women started to evolve, the intellectual messages regarding this relationship started to change. Now messages such as *Men and women are equal partners in a marriage* are starting to replace the old messages.

The problem with evolution is that it takes time. It can take time to change beliefs and intellectual messages. People can get stuck holding on to old messages, even in modern times. For example, even though the roles of men and women in society are evolving, people are still struggling to find a balance that both genders can be satisfied with. Both genders are still having trouble letting go of the old messages that told them women were responsible for all the cooking, housework, and child raising. Women still have a tendency to take on most of the responsibility for the household and child-care chores. And men let them do it. Although couples have a lot of conflicts over this issue, it is hard for them to evolve their intellectual messages and agree on new messages that both genders will be satisfied with.

The intellectual messages tribes teach their members are often subtle and difficult to recognize. These messages become so ingrained that they become part of our subconscious. We may not realize that we believe these messages, and we may even deny that we believe them if we are confronted with them, but they are part of our belief systems nonetheless. For example, you inherit your judgments about gays and lesbians from your tribes. You may not realize that you have these judgments because many people now believe it is wrong to have them. If someone asked you if you were homophobic, you'd say no. But if you are in a restaurant and see two gay men at the next table holding hands, you may be disgusted that they are displaying affection toward each other in public. If you are being honest with yourself, you will recognize the fact that although you deny it, you are really not totally accepting of gay people. You are still holding on to certain tribal messages about gays.

We all have an unlimited number of intellectual messages we believe in. All of our different tribes have been teaching us these messages since we were born. These messages become deeply entrenched in our intellects, and frequently we don't even consciously realize we believe them. It's as though they've become patterned into the neuronal pathways in our brains and have become a part of us. These messages can be healthy and regenerative. But they become a problem if they cause us to make choices that are harmful for us. As you are working on healing yourself, you will want to start identifying the unhealthy intellectual messages your tribes have taught you. You cannot afford to hold on to any tribal messages that do not support your individual health and inner peace. Once you have started identifying these messages, you can work on evolving them and replacing them with healthier messages.

▶ EXERCISE: Identify the tribes you belong to. Think about your family tribe, your friend tribes, and your work tribes. Notice your political, religious, ethnic, and racial tribes. Also observe your local, regional, and national tribes. Identify the tribes you belong to because of your beliefs and hobbies.

▶ EXERCISE: Pay attention to how you feel about each of your tribes. Do they facilitate healthy energy flow for you, or do they make you feel out of balance? Do you dread spending time with members of your tribes, or do you get excited about them and look forward to seeing them? After you spend time with them, how do you feel? Are you exhausted or energized? How do your tribes make you feel about yourself? Do they make you feel accepted and supported, or do they make you feel inadequate and uncomfortable?

▶ EXERCISE: Pay attention to the intellectual messages that the members of your tribes believe in. Ask yourself how these messages fit into your life. Are they healthy and regenerative, or do they lead you to do activities that are unhealthy for you? Do they support your inner peace, or do they make you think that there is something wrong with you?

▶ EXERCISE: Investigate the way people in different tribes and different cultures have lived throughout history. Watch movies and television shows and read books to gather your information. Also go to museums, and talk to older people about what life was like in the past.

Identify the different intellectual messages people are taught by their various tribes. Look for messages about how they should look, act, think, and talk. Observe how those messages vary among tribes. Notice how strongly tribal messages affect the members of the tribe. See how, throughout history, people have sacrificed their individual health for the sake of their tribal beliefs.

Observe how people at different times in history lived their day-to-day lives in different ways. For example, as you watch a movie set in the

THE INTELLECT

1800s, observe the ways people did their daily chores and notice how much more manual labor was required to survive compared to now. You can understand, when you see how hard life used to be, how we got into the habit of believing that life has to be hard. Then watch a movie about people living today, and you can see how life has become easier with all the new machines and technology. As you recognize the changes, try to appreciate the idea that life doesn't have to be so hard anymore.

Unhealthy Intellectual Habits

To bring your intellectual activity into balance, you will need to do more than simply tell yourself, *I will stop thinking all my unhealthy intellectual messages now*. Nothing makes the intellect more hyperactive than when you try to shut it down. That is what happens when many people try to meditate. Their objective is to focus on only one specific thought or to let go of their thoughts altogether. But when they try to do this, their intellects can fight back and get even busier and more intense than before.

If you find that meditation helps calm your intellect, continue doing it. But if it doesn't work for you, don't worry. You can use another approach to calming your intellect—one that involves working with your intellect and your emotions at the same time to bring them into balance together. The process of working with both sides of the emotion/intellect balance at the same time will make the process of calming your intellect much more successful than trying to work with your intellect all by itself.

The first step in this process of calming your intellect is to pay close attention to it and to all the thoughts that it is thinking. Imagine your intellect on the intellectual treadmill, obsessing on whatever thought is currently in your head. Notice how you get stuck on that thought and think it over and over again. Recognize how difficult it is to pull yourself off the treadmill and observe your intellect. It is difficult to change your perspective and say to yourself, *I'm going to ignore this thought now and think something else*. It's as though the magnet under the treadmill holding your intellect in place is so strong that your intellect can't break away from it and get off.

Your goal now will be to use your intellect to observe itself while it is walking on the thought treadmill. Imagine pulling part of your intellect away from the strong gravity field of the magnet under the treadmill. You are now going to use that part of your intellect to step back and observe the part of your intellect that is still on the treadmill. Instead of just focusing on the thought that has you on the treadmill, you are going to focus on the fact that your intellect is thinking the thought and that it is on the treadmill.

For example, after you see your son's not-so-stellar report card, the thought that has you on the thought treadmill may be: *I wonder if my son is stupid or lazy; maybe he'll be a failure in life.* You may have spent the last hour worrying and thinking that same thought over and over again. Now you want to step back and observe yourself on the thought treadmill thinking about your child's grades and his future. Instead of thinking about his grades, you will use your intellect to figure out what you have been thinking about. You may think, *Wow, look at my intellect thinking about my son's grades and his future. I see how it is on the treadmill and just keeps thinking the same thing over and over again.*

This will satisfy your intellect because it will be happy to still be working on thinking something. But as you pull it off the treadmill and instruct it to observe itself, you give it something to think about other than the thought it was originally obsessing over. This is the first step in teaching it how to get off the thought treadmill so it can rest.

To pull your intellect away from the thought treadmill, you will need to start observing yourself very closely. You will want to start listening to all the thoughts going through your head throughout the day. When you are alone doing your household chores or exercising or watching television, you will need to listen to all the thoughts that you are thinking. You can write these thoughts down in a journal if you want to, to help focus your mind on them. Otherwise, you can just pay attention and note them to yourself.

THE INTELLECT

When you are with other people, you will want to listen to the words that you speak and you will want to watch the actions that you take. Your words and actions are based on your thoughts, and they will give you hints about what you are thinking. Be as diligent about watching and listening to yourself as possible. This will help you identify all the intellectual messages going through your head.

As you become more aware of your thoughts, you will want to start identifying the unhealthy thought patterns that your intellect has a tendency to get stuck in. The work of identifying these unhealthy thought patterns will keep your intellect busy, but it will be a healthier busy than when it gets stuck on the treadmill thinking one specific thought. And it will help in the process of pulling your intellect off the treadmill altogether.

There are four unhealthy thought patterns you will want to watch for: planning, worrying, regretting, and judging. There are probably other unhealthy thought patterns, but working with these four is usually enough to help most people relax their intellects. If you find another one that is problematic for you, add it to the list.

The first unhealthy intellectual pattern you will want to watch for is excessive planning. You are planning whenever you make specific goals or arrangements regarding how you would like things to turn out in the future. There are short-range plans and long-range plans. Short-range plans include shopping lists and daily schedules; long-range plans involve our future dreams, such as what our children will be when they grow up. Planning in and of itself is not an unhealthy thing. In fact our world would be rather chaotic if no one ever made any plans. We need to make plans to get things done and to make it to appointments on time.

The problem with planning comes when the intellect gets on the planning treadmill and can't get off. One thing that can happen is that people can obsess over their plans so much that they lose the ability to appreciate what is going on in the present moment. They may be preparing for a major event, such as a wedding or Christmas, or planning smaller things, such as daily schedules. No matter how big the event is, the same thing can happen. They try to cover every detail so nothing will go wrong. They want things to be perfect, and they think that if they can plan well enough, they will be prepared for all contingencies.

The problem is that all their planning gets them trapped on the thought treadmill. They put all their energy units into their plans, so they aren't able to look around and experience their life fully in the present moment. A perfect example of this is with the Christmas holiday. Many people get caught up in planning the shopping, gifts, parties, decorations, and so on. By the time Christmas is over, they feel frazzled, exhausted, and empty. All their energy went into planning and carrying out the plans, and they didn't have time to stop and enjoy the season.

Another thing that can happen when you get caught up in excessive planning is paralysis. You can get so caught up in your plans that you can have a hard time taking action. For example, if your dream is to build your own house, you may spend years thinking about your plan, looking at different floor plans, deciding how many bedrooms and bathrooms you want, and so on. If you get too caught up in your plans, you may get so bogged down on the thought treadmill that you never actually get around to building your house. You are essentially using all your energy units to make your plans, and you don't have any left to put into your actions.

There is another problem with planning. Frequently life doesn't follow our plans. No matter how right your plans may seem, there is always a chance that things won't work out the way you thought they would. And you never know which plans will work out and which won't. While it is natural to make short-range and long-range plans, they aren't written in stone, and the outcome may end up being something you could never have imagined in your wildest dreams. When things don't work out the way you had wanted them to, it can be very hard to accept the loss and move on. People tend to deal with the loss of their plans in one of two ways. Either they try to use their intellects to control the outcome or they go into denial mode.

THE INTELLECT

A common example of a situation in which people try to control the outcome of their lost plans is when parents have a child who doesn't turn out the way they had planned. Parents invest so much time and energy into their children that it's natural for them to imagine what their children's lives will be like. They dream about what careers their children will have, how they will go fishing or bake cookies together, and how their children will get married and have children of their own. The problem comes when reality doesn't follow the script. Maybe their child has an illness and will never be the person his parents imagined he would be. Or maybe the child decides to drop out of college and join a rock band instead of being a doctor as they had planned.

It can be very tempting for parents to try to force their children to follow their plans. They may try to shame their child into doing what they want, or they may use money to bribe their child into doing what they want. They may say, "I'll buy you a new car if you finish college." The problem with this is that the child has the right to live his own life and make his own decisions. If parents try to control their child's life, they are putting a lot of energy into a plan that isn't really theirs to make. Sure, with the right bribe you can probably get your child to do almost anything, but it is unhealthy to block your child's personal growth in order to make your own plans work out. And it is likely that you will damage your relationship with your child because of your controlling approach.

You may have dreams for yourself that didn't work out. Maybe your life isn't going the way you had imagined it would. Maybe you have the job you dreamed of, but it is too exhausting or you really don't like it. It is tempting to try to use your intellect to find a way to keep pushing yourself to stay in your job and make your plan work even if this isn't the healthiest route for you to take.

The problem with forcing plans is that fighting reality takes a lot of energy units. As much as you would like to have things work out a certain way, you are going to squander a lot of energy trying to control the situation if it isn't meant to work out. You may be able to hold things together for a while, but over time you are going to feel your energy dwindle. Remember that you only have a limited amount of energy units to work with every day. If you waste those energy units trying to force something that isn't going to work out, you won't have any energy left to help you switch gears and make a new plan.

Some people go into denial when their plans don't work out. They use their intellects to lie to themselves and to the people around them, and they pretend that everything is still going forward as planned. For example, a father may be in denial that his son is gay, or a wife may be in denial that her husband is an alcoholic. The problem with this approach is that continually denying your reality uses up a lot of energy units. You have to constantly be controlling your thoughts so they don't let the real truth come through. The more energy units you spend on denying your reality, the less you will have available to help you make new plans.

Many times people make plans according to what their tribes tell them they should do. If your family tribe expects you to give everyone expensive birthday gifts each year, you can get caught up in trying to meet that expectation. This is a nice idea, but what if you are having financial trouble and can't afford to buy so many gifts? It can be hard to give up plans that your tribe expects you to follow. You can have a sense of failure, and you may be afraid of how your tribe will react when you don't come through for them. Will they reject you because you can't fit in? Your tribal messages can compel you to hold on to unhealthy plans.

You will now want to catch yourself when you are on the intellectual treadmill caught up in excessive planning. Watch for times when you are planning so much that you miss out on experiencing the present moment. Watch for situations in which your plans aren't working out and you are either trying to force the situation to work or denying that the situation isn't working.

For example, imagine that you are getting married next month. You may be totally consumed by all the plans. There are so many details that need to be taken care of before weddings that couples can get swept up in the long lists of things that need to be accomplished. You may have your days scheduled from morning to night with no time off to rest. Because of all this intellectual activity, you may have trouble relaxing in the evening. Your intellect can't get off the intellectual treadmill. When you lie down to go to sleep, your mind may still be racing, trying to remember details you have forgotten. Your family and friends may make comments about how stressed out you seem, and you may find yourself getting in arguments with your fiancé over wedding details.

Your goal is to pull yourself away from the planning treadmill and observe your intellect as it is going through its lists and plans. Now you are changing your perspective on the situation. You are still using your intellect, but it has a slightly different job to do. Instead of focusing on the details of the plans, your intellect is focusing on the fact that it is planning. You may now find yourself thinking, *Look at how my intellect is going through all its lists. Look at how it is trying to figure out the seating arrangements for the reception dinner. Look at how it is trying to figure out where to seat Grandma and Aunt Sylvia so they don't argue. I can see how busy my intellect is today, and the thought pattern I am stuck in is planning.*

You will want to do the same observation technique when your intellect is stuck on the treadmill trying to deal with plans that didn't work out. For example, maybe you have always dreamed of being a nurse, but once you got through nursing school and started working in a hospital, you discovered that you hate it. As you watch your intellect on the treadmill, you see that it is running the same thought loop over and over in your head: *I hate this. I hate this, but I make good money. What else could I do to make this much money? Maybe if I try working the night shift I'll like it better. Maybe if I try working in a different department in the hospital I'll like it better.* You will want to use your intellect to observe itself and notice the fact that the thought loop running through your head involves what you can do when your plans aren't working out.

Once you are able to identify yourself being caught up in excessive planning, you are ready to move on to the next step of relaxing your intellect. This step involves working with your emotions. Take a moment to stop and remember where intellectual hyperactivity begins. Remember that we are born feeling our emotions in a healthy way, but as we grow up, adults teach us to suppress our emotions and use our intellects to analyze and control ourselves. When we have an uncomfortable emotion, we get in the habit of thinking thoughts instead of feeling the emotion. We get taught to use our intellects to hold the lids on our emotional organs tightly closed. When you catch your intellect acting in a hyperactive fashion, you can almost guarantee that at the root of that hyperactivity is an unfelt emotion.

When you catch your intellect obsessing about your plans for the future, you can assume that beneath the plans is fear. Remember that the unknown of the future frequently causes us to feel fear. Instead of feeling our fear about the unknown, we learn to try to control things by thinking with our intellects. You may also have sadness or anger to feel in addition to the fear. You may be sad over your lost dreams. Or you may be angry because things didn't work out the way you had wanted them to.

When you find your intellect stuck on the planning treadmill, focus on letting your body feel the emotions that are sitting underneath your plans. At the same time, keep reminding your intellect that the reason it is obsessively planning is to avoid your emotions. Remind yourself that most of the work the intellect needs to do to make plans takes only a few minutes and energy units, and the rest of the time you spend on the intellectual treadmill reviewing those plans is wasted time and energy.

It might take some time to allow your emotions to flow. Do the exercises in the emotion chapter if you need to use them as triggers. As your body gets used to feeling emotions again, you will find that your intellect will start to relax. You will find that the process of feeling your emotions over a situation is always more healthy than getting stuck on the intellectual treadmill.

THE INTELLECT

You will find that some plans and dreams are harder to let go of than others. Some plans are more stuck in your intellect than others are. You may have had a dream that started when you were really young, or you may have a tribal message telling you that a certain plan is especially important for you. For whatever reason, some plans can seem so important that even if they aren't working out, you can have a lot of trouble letting them go.

You will find that the more attached you are to a certain plan, the more emotions you will likely need to feel before your intellect can stop obsessing over that plan. Don't judge the amount of time you need to work on this process of feeling your emotions associated with a certain plan. Keep feeling your emotions, and you will find that eventually you will be able to let go of your most deeply entrenched plans. You will also clean your emotional basement of all the emotions that had been associated with those plans. As you bring your emotions and intellect into balance, you will free up energy units to put toward new plans.

The second unhealthy thought pattern is worry. Worrying is the thinking and analyzing you do when you are looking at something unknown in the future that gives you fear. Instead of feeling your fear, you use your intellect to tell stories about the scary situation. Maybe you are feeling fear over the fact that you don't have enough money to pay the rent next month. Instead of feeling the physical emotion of fear, your intellect gets on the intellectual treadmill and thinks about the situation, wondering where you will get the money and what will happen if you don't.

Or maybe you are lying in bed worrying because your teenager is still not home at one o'clock in the morning. It can be easy to get on the intellectual treadmill and worry about where your child is. You may be imagining things that could be happening to him: *Was he in an accident? Was he hurt? Did he just get a flat tire? Why doesn't he answer his cell phone?* You may have fear because you don't know what happened. Or you may have anger because he has done this before and knows it upsets you. But instead of feeling your emotions, you are on the worry treadmill, analyzing and thinking about the situation.

If your sister is injured in a skiing accident and you are waiting to know if she will survive, you may have a lot of fear. But instead of feeling your fear, you may find your intellect getting on the worry treadmill. Your intellect will try to figure out how the accident happened, and it will want to get all the details of her medical condition. It may analyze the health-care workers and try to figure out if they are doing their jobs correctly. It will think about the future and what may happen if she doesn't survive. All the thinking that you do in this situation is worrying.

When you first start paying attention to your intellectual habits, it can sometimes be difficult to differentiate between doing basic problem solving and worrying. You may wonder how you will know when your thoughts stop being useful and when they become worries. The answer is that your intellect usually does its problem solving immediately after it becomes aware that there is a problem to solve. And usually all your valuable problem-solving thoughts will only take a few minutes to process. The rest of the time you spend thinking and analyzing is spent worrying. If you are thinking the same thoughts over and over again, you are worrying.

Worrying is like planning. It is an unhealthy intellectual habit that wastes energy. It is not beneficial or healthy for you to worry. You can approach worrying the same way you deal with planning. Recognize that there is probably an emotion underlying your worrying. Fear is often at the root of what you are worrying about, just as it is often at the root of your plans. Sadness and anger may be there as well. When you catch yourself worrying, feel the underlying emotions at the root of your worries. Remind your intellect that your worrying is a habit you've learned in order to suppress your emotions. As you learn to feel your fear instead of worrying, you will find that you won't lose so many energy units when you come up against the unknown of the future.

The third unhealthy intellectual habit is regret. You may look back at something you did to hurt another person and regret it. Maybe you were a bully in high school, and now you wish you hadn't acted so cruelly. Or maybe you are a parent and last week you yelled at your kids, and now you regret it. You can also have regrets about choices you've made that ended up causing yourself pain. You may look back and regret that you got involved in a certain relationship. Or you may wish you had moved to a city that suited you better than the one that you chose.

You can also regret things other people said or did that hurt you. You may regret that your boss fired you from a job you really liked. You may regret that your friend started a rumor about you. Or you may regret that you were abused as a child.

Whenever you look back and find yourself thinking about something that still bothers you about the past, whether you did it or someone else did, you are regretting. Regrets are your intellect's way of analyzing the situation and trying to come to some type of resolution over it. Your intellect will get on the thought treadmill and tell the same story over and over again, trying to come to terms with it. It may play with the story, trying to imagine a different outcome. Or your intellect may judge the situation and think, *That person was so terrible to do that awful thing to me!*

A common cause of regrets is suppressed emotions. It is natural to find our emotions being triggered during intense life situations, but we usually don't let ourselves feel those emotions fully. Instead, we get taught to suppress them and to put them into our emotional basements. We think that if we stop ourselves from feeling things too deeply, we will be able to move on and forget the past more easily. The problem is that you can't truly let go of the past if those emotions are still sitting in your body. They end up festering inside you and keeping you attached to your memory of the past, as much as you would like to let it go.

When you don't let yourself feel your emotions, you get stuck on the regret treadmill and bring your energy flow out of balance. Rather than thinking about the past, it is much healthier to feel the emotions that are in your emotional basement. You will find that the process of feeling your emotions will give you more energy than getting stuck on the intellectual stories about what you regret. You will find that as you clean out your emotional basement, you will be able to let go of the past for once and for all.

If you find yourself regretting a situation from the past, you will need to do the same thing you would do if you found yourself planning and worrying. For example, you may find yourself regretting a past marriage. Now instead of just looking back and judging all the failings of your ex or obsessing about how you might have been able to do things differently, you will want to first step back and observe your intellect as it runs on the thought treadmill, thinking one thought after another about the marriage. See yourself thinking all those thoughts, and be aware that those thoughts are regrets. As you are watching yourself, you may find yourself thinking, *Oh, look at how my intellect is stuck in its regrets about the past. The story I tell myself about the time my ex had an affair is a regret. The thought I always have when I wonder what I could have done differently to save the marriage is a regret. Look at how all these thoughts are regrets.*

Then focus on feeling the emotions triggered by the situation. It may take some time to clean out the room in the emotional basement that holds the emotions from the situation, especially if you've held on to a specific regret for a long time or if the situation was especially intense for you. You can't judge the amount of time it takes to feel the emotions connected to a specific regret. Have faith that with time, you will work through the emotions connected to the situation and come to a sense of peace over it.

The fourth unhealthy intellectual habit is judgment. Judgment is the thought process we use to evaluate the quality of things: good or bad, right or wrong. There is a broad range of judgments we all make every day. We wake up, look outside, and judge the weather as being good or bad. We look at ourselves in the mirror and judge our appearance as being attractive or ugly. We look out the window and compare our lawn to the lawn next door. We go to work and judge the way our coworkers look and act.

We are constantly judging ourselves and others. We judge every aspect of our lives. We judge ourselves and our worthiness to be accepted by our tribes. We judge the other people in our tribes, and we try to decide if what they are doing is acceptable. We judge the state of the world around us and decide whether it is good or bad.

We start judging in childhood. As our intellects are developing and we start being able to understand what people around us are saying, we are taught to judge. The adults around us teach us which judgments should be important to us. As we grow up, our tribes are constantly giving us new judgments to believe in. Judgments are one of the most powerful tools that tribes have for controlling their members. Each tribe has its own set of judgments it chooses to believe in. The tribe uses these judgments to let its members know how they can fit in. For example, if a tribe makes the judgment that pierced tongues are beautiful, people with pierced tongues will be appreciated by the tribe. If a tribe judges that drinking alcohol is a sin, people who drink alcohol may be shunned by the tribe.

As children grow up, they learn their tribes' judgments. Because they are motivated to fit in, they start internalizing those judgments. In the beginning they need the adults around them to tell them which judgments to make, but with time no one has to remind them, and they remember the judgments naturally, without any reinforcement.

One of the most common and powerful judgments children in all tribes learn to make is that feeling their emotions is bad or dangerous. This judgment starts children on the path of blocking their emotions. In the beginning they need reinforcement from the adults around them to block their emotions, but with time they do it without being told to.

Although making judgments helps you fit into your tribe, the process of judging is unhealthy. It brings your energy out of balance.

It is tempting to think that your judgments are important and that you need to hold on to them. But in reality, all they do is put you on the intellectual treadmill and hold you hostage there. Judging is only healthy when you are on a jury or doing a job that requires you to make judgment calls based on your experience. Otherwise, judgment is an unhealthy thought pattern.

We may think we have the right to judge other people and say that they need to change. The problem is that you can never change another person, no matter how much you would like to. There is only one person you can change—yourself. If you try to make other people change, they may seem to be complying with your wishes, but true change can only occur when they are motivated to change for themselves. If they don't really want to change, eventually they will return to their old habits or start to resent you for controlling them, and that will be unhealthy for your relationship.

Some of the most harmful judgments are those that we make about ourselves. People constantly evaluate themselves and decide they are not good enough. You may think you are not attractive enough, thin enough, smart enough, rich enough, or successful enough. You will judge yourself according to the values you are taught by your tribes. You will use those values as the standards by which you compare yourself to other people. If you don't meet the standard that your tribe has made for you, you will judge yourself as inadequate. Holding on to this type of judgment is unhealthy, and it blocks your energy flow.

Having the goal of nonjudgment does not mean that we should just ignore our personal responsibility for following societal laws. We should never deliberately hurt other people. We can't allow people to murder each other or steal from each other or abuse each other. The goal of nonjudgment is not to shirk responsibility but to help us avoid wasting our energy on unhealthy activities. Our energy would be much better spent healing ourselves and helping others rather than judging.

Your goal is to become so nonjudgmental that you judge nothing and no one, including yourself. You don't want to judge your friend's

THE INTELLECT

bad choice in men. You don't want to judge your coworker's new haircut. You don't want to judge the state of politics or the government. You don't even want to judge a murderer you read about in the newspaper. The time you spend on the intellectual treadmill judging is wasted time. The energy units you put into judging are wasted energy units, and you will never get them back.

People frequently judge because they think there is something wrong that should be changed. But judging something will not change it. It is much healthier to stop judging and instead feel your emotions. For example, you may be watching the news and listening to stories about all the terrible things happening in the world. You may get angry and think, *What kind of terrible person could do that awful thing to someone else?* That is a judgment. Your intellect is deciding that the person on the news is bad. Remember that unless you are on a jury or doing a job that requires judgments based on your experience, you don't want to waste your energy units on judging.

Rather than judge, a healthier approach is to feel all the emotions that the situations you are judging trigger in you. This will change the quality of your experience. It will be much more beneficial for your energy flow. You may have to put some time and energy units into stopping and feeling the emotions that were at the root of your judgments. But later on when you've cleaned out your emotional basement, you will have many more energy units available to work with. You can use your increased energy to do things to make the world a better place. Letting your emotions flow and acting on issues that upset you is a much healthier way of dealing with the world than sitting on your couch and spending your time thinking about what a terrible world it is.

When you are working on identifying your judgments, you will find that they are often mixed in with your plans, worries, and regrets. Part of the reason you can get caught up in those other thought patterns is because you have an underlying judgment that complicates them. For example, your judgment may be that to have a good Christmas party, you need all the right decorations, food, gifts, and music. You may catch yourself planning excessively and worrying about your Christmas party because your judgments tell you you'll be a bad host if you don't do things the right way.

When you find yourself regretting something from the past, you may find that you have a judgment attached to that regret. For example, maybe you built your house in an area that you were told would never flood. But maybe the first flood in a century came along and flooded your house. You may find yourself judging the experts who told you this couldn't happen as jerks or idiots. Every time you think about the situation you may visualize those experts and judge them. In this situation, simply feeling your anger about it won't be enough; you also need to work on letting go of the judgments that are holding you attached to your regrets.

How do you let go of judgments? The first thing you will want to do is identify your judgments the same way you identify your plans, worries, and regrets. Only when you are aware of them can you let them go. Watch your intellect as it gets stuck on the intellectual treadmill, and identify when it is judging. Once you have identified a judgment, there are two exercises that are especially helpful in letting it go.

The first exercise for letting go of your judgments is to change your perspective on the situations you are judging. Step back and observe them and see them from a different viewpoint. For example, if you are looking at a picture of a scenic mountain view that you don't like, instead of saying, "That is an ugly picture," say, "That is a picture with mountains, trees, and sky." The process of saying the picture is ugly is judging it; whereas if you simply identify the elements of the picture, you are observing it and not judging it. Once you have observed the picture, you may feel a sense of anger or repulsion, but the physical experience of feeling anger and repulsion is different than judging it.

Another example would be if you were getting on a bus and you were on crutches because of a sprained ankle. Imagine that the woman getting on the bus in front of you took the last available seat, and now you have to stand in the aisle. You may think, *That terrible, selfish woman should have given me the last seat. Can't she see that I'm disabled?* You may find yourself focusing on how awful she is, and you may even think about all the terrible things you would like to do to her, such as hitting her over the head with your crutches. Recognize that the process of thinking that the woman is terrible and selfish is a judgment. Instead of judging her, your new goal is to look at the situation with a purely observational eye: *The woman with the red coat and blond hair was ahead of me in line getting on the bus. There was one seat available when we got on, and she sat in that seat. Now I am standing in the aisle. I have a sprained ankle, and I am feeling pain in my ankle because I am standing on it.*

Don't waste your time judging the woman on the bus as good or bad; instead, observe the facts of the situation. This can be hard to do because we are taught to focus so much on our judgments. You may even have trouble at first differentiating between judgments and observations. Remember that judgments are thoughts that compare things and evaluate whether they are good or bad, right or wrong. Observations are neutral, detached thoughts that are not dependent on a specific outcome. Observations review the facts without an agenda or a preconceived notion regarding what is right or wrong. When you observe something, you step back and see it from a wider viewpoint, a viewpoint that acknowledges that there are many sides to any situation. While your viewpoint may be the only one you currently see, as you observe you can appreciate that other viewpoints may be just as real and valid.

Instead of judging the woman on the bus as a terrible, selfish woman, step back and observe the situation and recognize that while she may seem selfish, maybe she has chronic pain, and although she looks healthy, she may be in severe pain herself. Or maybe she just found out that her father died, and she is in shock and doesn't notice how selfish she is acting. You don't know why she is doing what she is doing, so don't waste energy units on assumptions.

What you will notice when you focus on observing and not judging is that behind judgments are usually emotions that need to be felt. As you are stepping back from the judgment and observing, let your emotions flow. If you are angry at the woman on the bus, breathe the anger through your body. Remember not to project it onto anyone else. Remember that the process of feeling emotions is always healthier than getting caught on the intellectual treadmill.

You can use this exercise of stepping back and observing the situation not only with judgments but also with other intellectual stories you get caught up in. A good example of where this exercise is useful is on the subject of money. People frequently get on the intellectual treadmill worrying about money. They worry about not having enough, and they worry about where they should spend it. They judge that they are poor or that they are inadequate because they don't have as much money as other people do. There are countless stories and judgments that people make concerning money.

If you find yourself on the intellectual treadmill worrying and making judgments about money, step back and observe the situation from a different perspective. Try to back up far enough to see a broad overview of your life, as if you were up in a hot-air balloon looking down on yourself, your house, and your neighborhood. Now shift your perspective, and try to visualize your life in a totally different way, a way that you may not have seen it before. See your life as being based on energy flow. See how your energy flows into you and through you, and see how you spend your energy on activities and the people around you.

Now see money as a symbol of your energy flow. See that the money that comes into your bank account is part of your fluid energy system. The money coming into your bank account represents energy flowing into the system. See how your money expenditures are symbolic of your energy expenditures. What you spend your money on is what you spend your energy on. If you spend your money on your house and your cars, you are putting your energy into your house and your cars. If you spend it on your children, you are spending your energy on your children.

THE INTELLECT

Change your intellect's perspective to see money not only as a number in your bank account but also as part of the fluid energy flow in your life. See your money as a tool to help you manifest your energy flow into physical form. Recognize that you need to spend it in a way that is healthy for the system.

Remember that your physical body is the ultimate physical manifestation of your energy flow. Envision your energy flowing into your body and out of it again. While money is a symbol of energy flow, your physical body is the most vital physical aspect of your energy system. Instead of focusing on the fact that you don't have enough money, focus on how you can bring your energy flow into the healthiest balance. Focus your intellect on your whole system—including your energy, your body, and your life—rather than just focusing on your money.

As you take this new viewpoint, you may find alternate approaches to your financial problems that you hadn't previously considered. You may see different sources of money that you had previously missed. You may see that you have energy sources that don't obviously look like a dollar bill, but that can still help you meet your system's needs. For example, if you are having trouble paying your mortgage, as you step back and view the situation from afar, you may notice all the extra space in your house and realize that you can rent out a room to a friend who needs a place to live.

As you look at the situation with this new viewpoint, you may decide that you need to change the way you spend your money and your energy in order to make the system more balanced. Maybe you need to cut back on spending in areas you hadn't previously considered. As you step back and view the situation from afar, those areas may become clearer to you.

You may find that when you step back and observe the situation from a different viewpoint, you can't immediately see any different solutions for the problem. If your financial situation is tenuous, you may just have to wait awhile before you will know how things will turn out. When you are in the time of waiting, you will want to continue to work on both sides of the emotion/intellect balance. Continue to step back and see the situation from the broader perspective so that any new solution will become clear when it is available. Also feel your emotions while you wait. Remember that feeling your emotions is always healthier than allowing your intellect to run on the thought treadmill.

It may be hard to take your focus off your money or whatever unhealthy thought pattern has you stuck on the intellectual treadmill. But stepping back and observing the situation from another perspective will be much healthier for you than staying trapped on the treadmill. As you change your perspective and feel your emotions, you will start to free up energy units that you had previously been wasting. You will be able to use those energy units to make the healthy changes that are needed in your life.

The second exercise to help you let go of your judgments is to find a replacement message for them. This is especially helpful when you find yourself repeating a long-held judgment over and over again. For example, if you have a message that you have inherited from your tribe, it can be very difficult to let it go. Maybe you find yourself judging that you are a failure because you dropped out of college and because your family and friends are saying how terrible it is that you didn't finish the program. Although you know it is better for your emotional health to have dropped out because you weren't happy, you may continue to have that judgmental voice in your head reminding you that you are a failure.

When you identify a pervasive judgment, you may need to work on finding a new intellectual message to replace it. You may need to write the new message on a piece of paper and read it a hundred times a day at first, but with time you will be able to replace the old judgment with the new message. A new message for a person dealing with the judgment of dropping out may be: *I can't hold on to any judgment that is unhealthy for me, no matter how important my tribe thinks it is. I know that I would not have been happy finishing college and doing a job that made me miserable. That would not have been a healthy thing for me to do. If my tribe doesn't support my health, I can't worry about what they think about me.*

When you work on creating a replacement message, you aren't just trying to change a thought habit. You are also creating new neuronal connections in your brain. Research done over the last decade, using newer brain-imaging techniques, has shown that when you work on changing your thoughts, you change your brain chemistry. So when you work on thinking a new thought, you are changing it both in the nonphysical part of your intellect and in your physical brain.

When you are working to find a new intellectual message, don't just try to think happy thoughts. That is unrealistic. Instead, think of a new message that will be something you can believe in, something that is neutral and nonjudgmental, and something that focuses on regeneration rather than degeneration. For example, it is easy for parents to judge themselves as failures if their children have problems. If you are the mother of a child who has a drug addiction or another problem, it can be easy to blame yourself. You may judge yourself as a bad mother because you failed at raising a perfect child. Instead of telling yourself, *I am a bad mother because my child has problems*, find a new intellectual message that is nonjudgmental. It may be something like this: *I may have made what I think were mistakes when I was raising my child, but I am human and every human makes mistakes, and I can't judge myself for being imperfect. I did the best I could with the resources I had. I also need to remember that I can't judge my child's life. Every human has lessons to learn, and for my child, one of the lessons was to become a drug addict.*

The process of finding a new intellectual message will need to be individualized to each judgment you deal with. Sometimes you may need someone you trust to help you develop the most regenerative intellectual message. The message may change as you work through the judgment and start to see it differently. In the beginning you may focus on one aspect of the judgment, and later on you may find another aspect to work with.

As with all the other work you do with the intellect, as you start to believe the new intellectual message, you will probably also find emotions you need to feel as well. You may be angry and sad because you have been hurt by the old judgment, or you may feel fear as you imagine living with the new intellectual message. Feeling your emotions will help you let go of your unhealthy judgments and help solidify the new intellectual messages into reality for you.

Be aware that this concept of developing a new intellectual message is different from the idea of positive thinking. There has been a movement in the United States during the last forty years that has told people that if they think positive thoughts, they will have unlimited success and good health. The difference between the power of positive thinking and the exercise here is that when you do this exercise, your goal is not to put a positive spin on everything.

Note that the word *positive* is a judgment. Anything that makes comparisons is a judgment. It doesn't matter if the judgment is that something is good or that something is bad; it is still a judgment. The problem with good judgments is that if there is something good, there will have to be something bad to compare it to. For example, if there is a good child in a family, the other children in the family will know that they are not as good. Even if no one says it specifically, the good child and the bad children in the family know who they are. Another problem with judging someone as good is that you put him or her on a pedestal that can take a lot of energy to try to maintain. So although *positive* and *good* seem like nice concepts, they are not healthy from an energy standpoint.

There are some other problems when you try to use positive thinking to let go of your unhealthy intellectual messages. One problem is that if you have deeply entrenched judgments telling you how bad you are or how you can't change your life, simply thinking a positive thought won't be enough to dig deep down and reverse the deeply entrenched, unhealthy messages. You may say the positive thought over and over again, but the unhealthy judgments will still

THE INTELLECT

be there, deep inside you, working against the positive thought. Only when you acknowledge and work through your dark thoughts can you truly let them go.

Another problem with positive thinking is that if you are always trying to be positive, you won't be able to let your uncomfortable emotions of anger, sadness, and fear flow. You can't truly heal yourself if you don't embrace all aspects of yourself, even the painful, "negative" ones. Although positive thinking is an attractive concept, it actually works against healthy emotional flow and healthy energy flow.

It can take some time to relax your intellect, but as you work with your emotions and your intellectual messages, you will start to understand experientially how this works. With time you will find that your judgments and unhealthy thought patterns will start to loosen their hold on you. You will be able to bring your emotions and your intellect into healthy balance.

▶*EXERCISE: Practice different exercises to calm both your intellect and your body. Try the breath-work exercises from the chapter on emotions. Try yoga, meditation, or energy work such as Tai Chi or Qigong. If you find that these relaxation techniques are helpful for you, do them on a regular basis.*

If your intellect resists the above relaxation techniques, try other activities to help your intellect relax. Try activities such as gardening, painting, cooking, listening to music, walking, swimming, or spending time with children or animals. These activities allow your intellect and your body to stay active with a lower intensity of functioning than if you were doing something very intense. But at the same time, you can relax when you are doing these activities because your intellect and your body don't have to be on full alert. You don't want to force yourself to do things that aren't fun for you, so focus on things you enjoy doing. If you have trouble figuring out what to do, think back to your childhood and remember what you used to enjoy doing as a kid.

If you can't find any hobbies that are relaxing, you know you have a huge problem with a hyperactive intellect, and you will need to continue to work on finding relaxing activities while you also do the work on calming your unhealthy intellectual habits.

▶ *EXERCISE: To recognize your intellect's unhealthy habits, start paying attention to what your intellect is thinking about. Visualize it on the intellectual treadmill, and recognize the specific thoughts it is focusing on as it runs on the treadmill. See the magnet holding it in place on the treadmill. Then visualize yourself pulling part of your intellect away from the treadmill, and let it observe itself on the treadmill. Observe the details of the thoughts your intellect is obsessing about as it spends time on the treadmill.*

▶ *EXERCISE: Pay attention to every thought that goes though your mind. Break those thoughts into at least four categories: planning, worrying, regretting, and judging. There may be other categories, but these four will give you plenty of material to work with. Start to be a witness to what is going on inside your head. If you like to keep a journal, write the thoughts down. Otherwise, simply observe and identify your thought patterns. Do this as much as you can throughout the day.*

In the beginning you may need to be rather disciplined with this exercise. If you are sitting in church listening to the minister's sermon, you will want to notice the stream of thoughts going through your head. Some of them may be related to the sermon and others may be totally unconnected to religion. As you observe yourself, you will want to pull yourself off the thought treadmill and think, What is this thought I'm having? Is it a judgment? a plan? a worry? a regret?

If you find that you can't slow down enough to pay attention to your thoughts throughout the day, sit quietly and spend an hour doing this as a more organized exercise.

Also observe what you say and do, and identify which of the four thought categories are behind your words and actions. Are you saying something based on a judgment? Are you acting in a certain way because you are worrying, planning, or regretting?

THE INTELLECT

▶ EXERCISE: When you recognize that your intellect is spending excessive time planning, worrying, or regretting, try to recognize and feel the emotions triggered by the situation. For example, when people are planning and worrying, they commonly have fear to feel. Thoughts of regret cover the gamut of emotions festering in the emotional basement.

▶ EXERCISE: When you are working with your plans, worries, and regrets, recognize any judgments that you have associated with those thoughts. For example, you may be regretting something you did in the past because you judge that what you did was stupid. In addition to feeling your emotions associated with the regret, you will also need to let go of the judgment underlying the regret.

▶ EXERCISE: Observe all the judgments you make—good and bad. Do this while you are sitting quietly and meditating or when you are driving in your car or having a conversation with someone.

Observe all your judgments for an hour or an entire day or whenever you have time to do it. An example would be: . . . judged my hair as bad this morning . . . judged my neighbor as looking ugly . . . judged my coworker as being a good person when she brought me a doughnut . . . This exercise will help you get to know the part of your intellect that judges.

▶ EXERCISE: Look at your judgments and beliefs and try to see the opposite side of the issue. For example, if you think that capital punishment is bad, try to find the good side of capital punishment. Look at your beliefs on religion, politics, abortion, interracial marriage, and gay rights. Look at your judgments about people of different races and ethnicities, including whites, blacks, Native Americans, Hispanics, and Asians. Look at judgments you have made about your family members and acquaintances, especially when they have done things you judge to be bad. Try to see the opposite side of the judgment in each situation.

▶EXERCISE: Try to recognize a situation where you have tried to make someone change. See the judgment behind your expectation that they should change. See the outcome, and be honest with yourself about how your demanding them to change has affected your relationship with them. See how the action of changing that other person is based on judgments, and identify the judgments behind your actions. Also try to see the situation from the other person's viewpoint.

▶EXERCISE: Another simple way to bring your awareness to your judgments is to repeat a simple intention, such as I fully intend not to judge, once a day or as often as you need to. Focusing on the fact that you intend to let go of your judgments can help you recognize when you are thinking them.

▶EXERCISE: Recognize when you are judging yourself. It is as important to let go of judgments about yourself as it is to let go of judgments about others, and to let them go, you first have to recognize them.

▶EXERCISE: Recognize when you are judging your emotions. For example, if you are talking to a friend and something you talk about makes you sad or afraid, catch yourself blocking the emotion. Recognize the judgment that is preventing you from letting yourself feel the emotion.

▶EXERCISE: When you catch yourself judging a person or a situation, step back and observe the facts of the situation with neutrality and non-judgment. Simply observe the situation instead of judging it. Pull yourself back as far as you need to until you can see the situation from a new viewpoint. If needed, imagine yourself flying above the situation in a hot-air balloon. Retell the story of the situation from this new viewpoint. Feel the emotions that are triggered as you change your perspective on the situation.

THE INTELLECT

▶ EXERCISE: When you catch yourself being stuck on the intellectual treadmill saying a judgment or an intellectual message over and over again, find a replacement message to use instead. Remember that you don't just want to think happy thoughts, but you want to have a new message that is regenerative and nonjudgmental. Write the message down and read it as often as you need to until you make it real for yourself. Feel the emotions that are triggered as the new message becomes more real for you.

▶ EXERCISE: Observe other people's intellectual messages and judgments. When you are watching a movie or listening to the radio or talking to other people, identify their judgments. Do not judge the other people for what they say or do; you are only observing them so that you can understand unhealthy intellectual messages and judgments more clearly.

▶ EXERCISE: Patients with chronic pain frequently have a cycle of blocked emotions and intellectual hyperactivity that leads to muscle tightness and then pain. If you have chronic pain, watch for this cycle. Notice when your pain is being caused by tight muscles (or clenched jaws, if you have headaches). Then observe what is going on with your emotions and your intellect. If you can let your emotions flow and calm your intellect, you will be able to improve the muscle tightness and the pain.

5 Shame

As you are dealing with your intellect and judgments, there is another issue you need to deal with: shame. Shame is the feeling that you have done something bad, something that you shouldn't have done. It can be a sinking feeling in the pit of your stomach, and it can make you sweat or feel nausea, butterflies, or dizziness. You might feel embarrassed and find yourself blushing. You may have the desire to hide or disappear or cover something up.

Shame is an emotion. We experience it in a physical way in our bodies just as we would feel any other emotion. But while shame is experienced physically in our bodies, it is similar to depression in that it is not a healthy, regenerative emotion to feel. The fact that shame is experienced physically in our bodies is the only thing it has in common with the other emotions. Shame isn't a natural, healthy part of us as the four key emotions are. It originates from a different place than the healthy emotions do; therefore, we need to deal with it differently than we deal with the others.

Shame is different from the healthy emotions because instead of originating in the body, it comes from the intellect and from our judgments. We all have a tendency to make judgments. We judge ourselves, and we judge the people around us. We compare ourselves to the people around us and decide whether we are good enough to match up. Sometimes we decide that we are, but often we decide that we aren't. The physical feeling of shame originates from our judgment of ourselves.

Shame works in the opposite direction of the healthy emotions. The healthy emotions start from deep within you and flow to the outside, healing you as they flow. Shame, on the other hand, starts from your judgments and intellect on the outside of your emotional organ and turns in on you. It works as a lock that holds the lid on the emotional organ closed. Since the lid is closed, your healthy emotions can't flow out of the emotional organ as they should. Shame ends up blocking your emotional flow and energy flow, and it inhibits healing.

The experience of feeling shame starts for most people when they are very young. They learn it from the adults around them as they are being taught to control their emotions and conform to the rules of their tribes. The adults around them want them to control themselves to fit in. When children are doing something their parents don't want them to do, at first their parents say, "Don't do that. That is a bad thing to do." But because children's intellects aren't fully developed, they don't always understand or care about what the adults tell them to do. When you are one or two years old, you are still focused on life in a very basic way, and your complex thought patterns and neuronal connections are not developed yet. You may not understand what adults are saying when they say, "You are a bad child, and you shouldn't do that bad thing because . . . " Or you may not have a reference point to which you can compare their criticism of you. You may not understand or agree with their reasoning. Because of this, using a gentle voice to control a child often doesn't get the response that an adult wants.

If a gentle voice doesn't work to control a child, adults frequently get more dramatic and say "Shame on you" with a voice that lets the children know they are in trouble. The shame-on-you voice may be loud or low and menacing; the exact words and volume of the voice don't matter. What matters is the threat that comes with it.

The shame-on-you voice may be accompanied by a spanking or

other physical punishment if the adult can't control the child with the voice alone. The spanking reinforces the power of the voice. Sometimes only one spanking is all that is needed to give the voice power that lasts for the rest of a child's life.

Children recognize the danger in the shame-on-you voice, especially if it is reinforced with physical punishment. Their parents may not realize how intimidating that voice is, but children take it very seriously. Children know they need the approval of the adults in their lives for them to fit in to their tribes and survive. They intuitively know that if they make adults angry, they may end up being injured or forced out of the tribe, so they start to feel shame and start to control their emotions to fit in and be accepted.

This may sound rather dramatic to an adult, but try to remember what it was like when you were a little child and all your safety and comfort depended on the adults in your life. Those adults seemed so large and omnipotent. You wanted to stay on their good side to feel safe and secure. When they weren't happy, either because of something you had done or because of another issue in their lives, you sensed a lack of security in your world.

Try to remember a time when you felt shame as a child. Maybe you did something naughty, such as stealing a candy bar from the grocery store or having a tantrum in church because you didn't get your way. You probably didn't understand yet why stealing or tantrums were bad, but when the adults in your life used the shame-on-you voice, you felt the physical feeling of shame as you realized you were in trouble. You may have felt shock and a feeling of heaviness in your gut. You may also have felt fear. The physical feeling of shame acted to cement the judgment that you were bad into your belief system.

It may be hard for you to remember shame from your childhood because it often starts when children are so young that their intellects haven't developed enough to understand it yet. Parents start to shame their children when they are less than a year old. It's doubtful that many adults will remember much about those early days in their lives. This is part of the reason why shame is such a difficult problem to recognize and understand. It is a habit that becomes patterned into our bodies before we are even aware of it. After having this habit for decades, it can be hard to see it, much less heal it.

Our tribes use shame to control all types of thoughts and behaviors. One of the first things most children start to feel shame about is their emotions. The other things that are considered shameful depend on the judgments of your individual tribe. An example of a behavior that is commonly considered shameful in Western culture is the inability of children to sit still in class for long periods of time. There is a judgment that children are bad or sick if they have an incredible amount of energy and need to run around and play for many hours each day. This can lead to a serious conflict when they start school. There is little room in most schools for children to have freedom to run. Instead, they need to be compliant and sit quietly in their seats. Their teachers and parents tell them they are bad and shame them for not being quiet. The shame is compounded if children can't learn their school lessons quickly enough. Over time the shame and judgments become internalized, and children start to tell themselves that they are bad and unacceptable.

Another unfortunate tribal message that is fostered in our culture is one that tells children that fitting in and being compliant is more important than having curiosity and individuality. Adults may give lip service to curiosity and individuality, but in reality they shame children when those traits get in the way of the priorities of the tribe. If a child's curiosity makes her question tribal beliefs, she may be shamed into suppressing it. If her curiosity makes her ask numerous questions and the adults around her are too busy to stop and answer them, the adults may shame her as a way to shut her up.

If a child's individual interests don't fit in with the tribe's, he may be shamed into suppressing his interests. If a boy loves to sew, but lives in family that thinks sewing is a sissy hobby for girls, he may be shamed into hiding his interest in sewing. Every tribe has beliefs and activities they value, and if a child doesn't share those beliefs or doesn't want to do those activities, then he or she will likely be shamed into changing to fit in.

Tribes also teach people to be ashamed of things that are natural, healthy aspects of being human. Sex and other body functions are frequently considered shameful, and different tribes judge specific body traits as bad and shameful. If a tribe judges a specific physical trait as undesirable, people with that trait will be taught to be ashamed of having it. If a woman is voluptuous and belongs to a tribe that values skinny women, it is likely that she will feel ashamed of her shape.

Shame is the ultimate tribal control mechanism. As tribal members are continually shamed, they start to believe the messages their tribes want them to believe. We go through our lives believing these messages, even though we may not even realize we are thinking them. Your tribe keeps you under its control with the messages it teaches you and with the feeling of shame that backs up those messages.

For example, if a woman is married to an abusive husband, she may want to leave him, but she may feel a sense of shame for giving up on her marriage. If her tribe has taught her that divorce is a terrible sin, she will want to avoid a divorce at all costs. The sense of shame she has learned to feel over failing at marriage may cause her to hide the abuse and stay with her husband, even if her life is in danger. She is being controlled by her tribe's judgments and by her shame.

Everyone experiences shame, but each person deals with it in a different way. Some people feel shame in some situations but not others. They may not feel it when they are with people who are accepting of them, or they may not feel it when they are in situations where they feel safe and in control. But when they are in uncomfortable situations with people they don't trust or when they are doing something they are not comfortable with, they may feel shame and embarrassment.

Some people feel a constant sense of shame that is always very close to the surface for them. It can plague every aspect of their lives, and they can be paralyzed by it. These people find that every time they try to make changes in their lives, the shame blocks them from moving forward, and they may constantly think and talk about how inadequate they feel.

Some people have a deep feeling of shame but have learned to deny it. If you were to ask them about it, they would deny feeling shame, but at the same time, their behaviors are obviously shame based. Keeping secrets is a shame-based behavior. If you feel that you can't tell someone the truth, you may be acting out of a feeling of shame. And if you find that you avoid certain people and situations because they make you feel inadequate, you are probably acting out of shame.

Some people have learned to deal with their own shame by projecting it onto other people. Somehow they learned that if they say or do something to shame someone else, they may be able to avoid feeling shame themselves for a little while. The problem with this approach is that deep down you will still feel your shame. And when you hurt other people you can alienate yourself from them and end up feeling isolated and alone. You may get a short-term sense of relief from your shame when you hurt other people, but over time you will have even more shame because you've added the shame of hurting someone to your shame list.

This brings up the issue of guilt. In many instances, people refer to the word guilt when they are discussing the shame-like feeling you get when you harm other people. For our purposes the words shame and guilt can be used synonymously. The physical feelings you have when you feel guilt and shame are the same. It doesn't matter whether your feelings of shame stem from an act you committed to harm another person or whether you feel shame because you are being judged for the way you are. You still need to feel the physical sensations that come with both types of situations.

When you are working on healing your shame, you first need to be able to recognize it and feel it physically. The only way you can work through it is to know when it's there. You will want to feel the physical feeling of shame just as you would feel any of the other emotions.

You will want to spend some time recognizing what shame feels like for you. Do you blush? feel nauseated? get dizzy? Do you get a sinking feeling in the pit of your stomach? Or do you just have an uncomfortable feeling that you can't characterize? You won't be feeling it forever, but to work through it, you first need to be in touch with it.

You may find that you have trouble feeling the physical feeling of shame at first. Instead of feeling physical shame, you may catch yourself on the intellectual treadmill obsessing over the shameful situation. You may find yourself replaying the situation over and over in your mind like a broken record, trying to figure out what you could have done differently. Or you might be so ashamed about the situation that you try to banish it from your thoughts altogether.

If you can't physically feel shame at first, try to recognize situations in which you are judging yourself and situations in which it would be natural for you to feel shame. For example, you might feel shame if you were walking down the street and accidentally tripped and fell flat on your face in front of a crowd. Most of us would be embarrassed and feel some shame in this situation. You might find yourself blushing and wanting to get away from the crowd. You might judge yourself for being a klutz.

Another situation in which many people would feel shame would be during a meeting at work if their boss criticized them in front of their coworkers. In this situation you would likely have some physical symptoms of shame, maybe a sinking feeling in the pit of your stomach accompanied by a sense of nausea and a racing heart. You might find yourself blushing and you may want to escape from the meeting.

Pay attention to present-day situations and past situations that have triggered your shame. Write about those situations if that helps make them more real to you. You can also talk to someone who was there, to bring the details into clearer focus. Let yourself remember times when you said or did embarrassing things that you would rather forget about. Also let yourself remember things you said or did to hurt someone else. Feel the shame connected to all those situations.

After you have started to recognize and feel your shame, you can go on to the next step of the process. While you want to be able to acknowledge your shame, feeling it for weeks or months or years on end isn't going to help you heal it. Shame doesn't have the same healing effect that the healthy emotions have. If you get stuck feeling shame for extended periods of time, it will just paralyze you and block your energy flow.

Once you have acknowledged your shame, you will want to work on changing your perspective toward it. Instead of thinking you have shame because you are bad, see that shame is always rooted in a judgment. Instead of focusing on the shame itself, your new goal will be to recognize the judgment that is triggering it. Only when you can see the judgment behind your shame can you resolve it.

If you feel shame because you tripped and fell in front of a crowd, the judgment may be that you are clumsy or that you always need to be perfect. If your boss criticized you in front of coworkers, you may feel shame because you judge that you are bad at your job. Or maybe you don't believe you are bad at your job, but you judge yourself as weak because you allowed your boss to victimize you in front of your coworkers.

Shame is a very valuable tool to help you recognize judgments and tribal stories that are problematic for you. Only judgments that are important to you will make you feel shame. If there is a judgment other people believe in but you don't agree with, you won't feel shame over it. For example, if your boss makes the judgment that you are bad at your job, you will only feel shame if you believe that judgment. If you don't agree with that judgment and you know you are good at your job, you won't feel shame over it.

Once you recognize the judgment behind your shame, you can deal with the judgment the same way you would deal with any other judgment or intellectual message. For example, if when you were young you were repeatedly told what a bad child you were, you may have internalized the judgment that you are a bad person and don't deserve to be happy. Now you may feel shame whenever you start to feel joy or whenever you need something from someone, because you judge that you don't deserve it.

You can step back, see the situation from a new perspective, and create a nonjudgmental, regenerative replacement message. A new message in this situation may be: *I recognize that the judgment that I am bad comes from my childhood and that it makes no sense. I was a typical child who made some mistakes but had a good heart. I can see how my tribe used that judgment to make me conform. Everyone deserves to feel joy and to have their needs met. I deserve that just as everyone else does.* Every time you feel the uncomfortable feeling of shame and every time you judge yourself as bad, pull out the piece of paper and review the new intellectual message.

As you work on recognizing judgments that have caused you to feel shame, also pay attention to the emotions you are suppressing with that shame. For example, if you recognize how you feel shame because you have judged yourself to be bad, you may be angry and sad over how you've been hurt by your judgments. You may need to grieve over the situation that has hurt you.

You will find that the process of letting the healthy emotions flow will help the new intellectual messages you have created become more real to you. The combination of working on both the emotions and the intellect together is very helpful. Over time your shame will fade away, and it may recur occasionally, but you will be able to put it into perspective much more easily.

The last step in dealing with shame involves the type of shame triggered when you deliberately hurt another person. Most of us have deliberately hurt another person at some time in our lives. It may have been something such as making fun of another kid in school or stealing something from someone else.

The problem with deliberately hurting another person is that it is unhealthy for your energy flow. Even if you try to deny that it is a problem, you will hold what you have done inside your body, and you will block your energy flow. You need to work through what you have done to bring your energy flow back into balance.

First you need to acknowledge your shame over what you have done, even if it is something you have tried to keep hidden. Let yourself physically feel the shame if you can. If you can't feel it, at least acknowledge to yourself that you would normally feel shame in that situation.

Once you recognize that you feel shame, you need to identify the judgment behind the shame. If you've hurt someone, the judgment will likely be: *It is bad to deliberately hurt other people.* Unlike most other judgments, which are unhealthy, this is an example of one judgment that is helpful because it allows us all to live together peaceably. We can't live in peace if we deliberately hurt each other, so of course we should judge the process of deliberately hurting another person as bad. It is appropriate to feel shame when you deliberately hurt someone else.

When you have acknowledged your shame over hurting the other person, you will need to work to heal the shame. Although it is healthy to feel shame when you have done something to deliberately harm someone else, you won't help yourself or anyone else by getting stuck in that shame forever. If you hold on to your shame, you can become so uncomfortable with yourself that you can go into a state of numbness and denial over what you have done. When you are in that state of denial, it will be easier for you to continue to deliberately hurt other people.

When you catch yourself feeling shame because you have done something to deliberately hurt another person, you will want to try to access the healthier emotions brought up by the realization of what you have done. Maybe you have grief over what you have done. Maybe you acted out of anger or fear; if that is the case, you need to feel those emotions in a healthy way without projecting them. The process of feeling emotions is vital to healing your shame. You may also need to work on the intellect side of the emotion/intellect balance. Step back and observe the situation from a broader viewpoint. Look for things that caused you to do the shame-inducing act. You may identify unhealthy intellectual messages that you have been taught by your tribe that led you to do the thing you did. Create healthy new intellectual messages to replace the old ones.

Finally, you need to take action. If it is appropriate, you need to apologize to the person you have hurt. You may need to do more than just apologize. You may also need to take action to make up for the harm you have done. What you need to do will be different for each situation. If you deliberately said something cruel to your friend because you were mad at him, maybe you only have to apologize and that will be the end of it. If you manipulated the situation after your parents died so that you would get more of their inheritance than your siblings, you will have to apologize and give a fair amount of money to your siblings. From an energy standpoint, you have no choice but to make amends. If you don't do this, you won't be able to heal.

If your shame is caused by something you did to hurt someone in the distant past, the action step may be different than if you hurt someone recently. You still need to recognize your shame, even if it is over something that you did forty years ago. It will still be bothering you deep down on some level, even if you have tried to forget it. You will still need to recognize the judgment at the root of your shame and create a healthier replacement message, and you will need to feel the emotions triggered by the situation. But the action you need to take may be different, especially if the person you hurt isn't alive anymore. Perhaps you did something to hurt your sister when you were young, but now she is dead. You may still feel shame about the situation, but you won't be able to apologize. If you can't apologize to her in person, you will need to find a way to help someone else in her place. Maybe you will want to do some sort of charity work to make up for what you did in the past.

When you apologize and make amends, your goal is not to get the other person to forgive you. It feels good if the other person is willing to forgive you, but you shouldn't expect it. Once you have deliberately hurt another person, the deed has been done and there is no going back. That person has to work through her injury in her own time. You have created a drama, and she has to deal with her part of the drama in her own way.

She may forgive you or she may not, and you have to accept the outcome of the drama no matter what it is. The important thing for you to remember is that it is not healthy for you to deny what you did or to dwell in your shame forever. It is much healthier for you to face your shame and work through it. Then spend the energy you would have wasted in shame working to improve the world around you.

Shame can be a painful thing to deal with. We've all been taught by our tribes to feel it, but we've also been taught to not acknowledge it. It takes courage to face your shame. At first you may have trouble recognizing it and may want to ignore it, but if you are serious about healing yourself, you have no choice but to deal with it. You will find that as you work on your shame, you will start to find a sense of freedom and inner peace.

▶*EXERCISE: Try to recognize the physical feelings associated with shame. Remember an embarrassing experience you had in the past or recognize one that you are experiencing now, and let yourself feel your shame.*

Next identify the judgment that caused you to feel the shame. Then do the exercises from the intellect chapter to calm the judgment. Step back and see the situation from a different perspective. Create a nonjudgmental, regenerative message to replace the judgment. Write the new intellectual message down if you need to. Every time the feeling of shame comes up, bring out the new intellectual message and review it. At the same time you are working on calming the judgment associated with your shame, feel the healthy emotions triggered by the situation.

This process may take time, and you may need to repeat the steps many times a day at first, but the new intellectual messages will start to replace the old judgments, and your shame will fade.

▶ *EXERCISE: If your shame was caused by an act you did to deliberately hurt another person, you need to do the work in the exercise above, and finally, make amends. Remember that it is always healthier to face the shame you feel when you have deliberately hurt another person and work to heal it rather than to deny it and risk hurting them again.*

6 The Intuition

As you are working on healing yourself, you will need to figure out what choices are the healthiest for you. Should you rest more? Should you change your diet? Should you try a different medication? Every day there are news stories telling us about new treatments that have been found to be beneficial for different medical problems. There are so many options that it can get confusing. How do you decide what is right for you?

In addition to needing to make choices regarding medical treatments, you also need to make a number of lifestyle choices. Is your relationship with your spouse healthy for you? Should you change to a less stressful career? Are there other changes you need to make?

How do you figure out how to make the choices that will be the healthiest for you? Many people depend exclusively on their intellects to make their lifestyle decisions. The problem with this is that the intellect can get caught up in unhealthy tribal messages and judgments, and it can lead you in the wrong direction. It can get caught up in a belief that may be beneficial for someone else but not for you.

Instead of depending on your intellect to guide you in making your life choices, you will want to let another part of your inner self guide you. That part of you is called *intuition*. Your intuition is the voice or feeling inside you that lets you know what decision or what step would be most beneficial for you at any point in time. Your intuition may present itself to you as a voice in your head, a gut feeling, or another physical sensation. It may appear as a picture in your mind. It may even come to you in a dream. People refer to *women's intuition* as though only women have intuitive guidance, but it isn't exclusive to women. Men have it too. Some people refer to their intuitive messages as *gut instincts*. It doesn't matter what you call it. What is important is that you learn to recognize it and listen to it.

Your intuition may give you a long-term sense of what will happen next month or next year. But the work you will want to focus on is the short-term, present-moment information it gives you every day. The importance of your intuition is that it is your own personal advisor who is always ready to tell you what would be most beneficial for you. It is the voice of your inner self, and it always has your best interests in mind as it gives you guidance.

Where does your intuition originate? Does it take information from your physical surroundings? Does it take information from your past experiences? Does it get its guidance from God or your higher power? No one really knows the answer to those questions because our intellects can't see all the secrets of the universe. Most likely our intuitions take guidance from all those places: our past experiences, the physical world, and God.

The origin of your intuitive guidance doesn't really matter. Since no one can prove where exactly our intuitive guidance comes from, we may as well not waste intellectual energy trying to answer that question. The important thing to recognize is that the intuition sees a bigger picture than the intellect sees. It can sense things that may not make sense to our intellects. It isn't caught up in judgments and analysis the way our intellects are.

We've all had intuitive messages that we've followed. Mothers regularly have intuitive feelings about what their children need. An artist may have an intuitive feeling about what colors will work together in a picture she is painting. A police officer may have an intuitive feeling telling him to watch his back just a minute before someone comes up behind him with a knife. Most people can remember times in their lives when their intuitions gave them messages that helped them in times of need.

As you are working to recognize your intuition, you will need to understand how it is different from your intellect and your emotions. The intuitive voice is neutral and not emotional, judgmental, or analytical. It simply informs you about what the best thing is for you in this moment. It isn't afraid, and it isn't judging the situation as good or bad.

Although your intuition isn't judgmental or emotional, sometimes it can give you an intense sensation as it guides you. For example, you may be driving to work and feel strongly compelled to turn right at a stoplight that you would normally go straight through. At the light you may be thinking, *Why do I feel so strongly that I should turn here? It makes no sense because I'm going to go out of my way if I take this other route, and I'll be late for my meeting.* You may find out later in the day that the reason you were compelled to turn right was because you avoided a car accident on the next block. Now you understand why your intuitive message was so strong.

Frequently the intuitive message is very quiet and gentle. It may not communicate to you with drumrolls or fireworks. You may have a choice between two jobs, and one job will feel right, but the other won't. It may be hard to pin down exactly why you feel that way; you just know that's the way you feel. Your intuition is giving you its guidance, and it's your job to listen to it.

The problem with the intuition is that its messages often get lost between the over-active voice of your intellect and your uncomfortable emotions. Your intuition may tell you, *I should stop eating meat*, but your intellect may tell you, *I can't stop eating meat. My entire family eats meat, and I'd have to change the way I cook. That would be a lot of work, and my family wouldn't be happy. Besides, people need protein in their diets to be healthy.* Your intellect may find several reasons why you shouldn't follow your intuition. Your intellect tends to get caught up on the intellectual treadmill with judgments, plans, worries, and regrets. It also gets caught up in the tribal messages you've been taught.

At the same time that your intellect is analyzing what your intuition is telling you to do, your emotions may get triggered by your intuition's suggestions. Your intuition may guide you to do something that triggers your fear. If your intuition tells you to quit your job and try a new career, you may feel fear because you would be changing your life in a dramatic way and facing the unknown. You may hate your current job, but at least you know you have the security of a guaranteed income while you are working there. You don't have any guarantee about the unknown situation your intuition is guiding you toward in your new career.

It is natural to feel fear and other emotions when you face the unknown of what your intuition is guiding you to do. The problem comes when you suppress the emotions your intuition triggers in you. If you suppress your emotions, you block your energy flow and can become paralyzed and unable to move forward to follow the guidance your intuition gives you. It is much healthier for you to let your fear and other emotions flow. They become fuel that gives you energy to follow through on your intuitive guidance.

While the intuition is always guiding us to do things that are most beneficial for us, it may not always guide us to do things that are the easiest or most fun. Our lives weren't meant to be perfect and without pain. We are on the earth to learn lessons. Those lessons aren't always that fun or easy, but instead they tend to be challenging and difficult. Sometimes your intuition will guide you to a situation that you don't necessarily like, but there is a lesson you need to learn from it.

One example of a painful experience that your intuition may guide you into is an unhappy marriage. Maybe when you got married, everyone around you told you that the person you were marrying wasn't the right one for you, but your intuition drew you into that relationship anyway. Now many years later, you may look back at the marriage and wonder, *How can I trust my intuition when it led me into that bad marriage?* You may now be afraid to listen to your intuition because you figure that it has led you astray.

But you need to remember not to judge the experiences your intuition leads you into. As you look back on your bad marriage, you will likely recognize some important life lessons it taught you. You wouldn't have learned those lessons if you hadn't followed your intuition's guidance telling you to get married. And while you will usually be able to look back and understand why your intuition led you into a certain situation, this won't always be the case. You may not understand why your intuition draws you into some situations that are painful for you. You may just have to take the leap of faith that there is a reason for them, try to learn what you can learn, feel your emotions, and move on. It's easy to try to hold on to safety and security, but sometimes the safe way is also the way that blocks your energy flow. Our lives are not meant to be stagnant. We are meant to be continuously moving forward and growing. Sometimes growth is painful and scary, but with time that pain may also bring healing. Your intuition is the part of you that is guiding you to that healing.

Imagine your life as a journey. Your body is the car that takes you on that journey. Most people let their intellects drive their cars. Their intellects decide where they will go and how they will get there. The problem with this is that when you let your intellect drive, it tends to get caught up in unhealthy thought patterns that aren't beneficial for your body or for your inner peace. It might say, *Let's drive down this safe path and follow the route that everyone else is taking.* But the path that everyone else is taking may not be the right path for you.

Instead, you will want to let your intuition be the driver of your car. Your intuition is able to see the road ahead with much better insight. Your intellect may not always understand why your intuition chooses the path it does because the intellect can't always see the big picture the way your intuition can. But your intuition always knows the best path for you to take.

Your intellect may fight losing control of the steering wheel to your intuition, but you will want to move it out of the driver's seat and give it a different job. You will want it to take over the work of the computer or the GPS in your car. When your intuition tells you where to go, you will want to have your intellect take its instructions and figure out how to get there. For example, if your intuition tells you that you should try eating Thai food, it is your intellect's job to find out where the local Thai restaurant is and how to get there. It isn't your intellect's job to analyze the situation to try and figure out if eating Thai food is a good idea.

The intellect has trouble moving out of the driver's seat. Your intuition may guide you into an unknown, scary neighborhood that your intellect sees as a bad thing. It may fight your intuition and take you on a detour into what looks like a safer neighborhood with fancy houses and nice lawns. Your intellect may think that it was really smart, helping you avoid the pain and fear of the unknown.

But the problem with the detours our intellects bring us on is that they come with their own learning experiences. There are painful lessons to learn even in the neighborhoods with fancy houses and nice lawns. And many times you will find that the detour your intellect thought was so smart will eventually come to a dead end, and you'll just have to get back on the original path again anyway. So you may as well cut the extra time and energy expenditures that your intellect tries to tempt you into and let your intuition streamline your life. Learn the lessons that your intuition tells you are important, and save your leftover energy for some fun.

If your intuition is the driver of your car and your intellect is the GPS, your emotions should be the fuel for your car. If you try to block them, your car will stall. Blocked emotions can also work like roadblocks or potholes; they will hold you back and prevent you from moving forward. But if you allow them to flow in a healthy way, they will give you energy and support your forward movement. If your intuition tells you to drive through that scary neighborhood but you don't let yourself feel your fear, you won't be able to move forward. Instead, you will be stuck feeling paralyzed. Your paralysis and blocked emotions will block your energy flow, and you may never get the chance to realize how wonderful things are in that unknown neighborhood.

You can use your intuition to help you answer any question that is troubling you. It will tell you the diet and exercise regimen that is right for your body. It will tell you if you should stay home and rest on Saturday night or go out to the party you were invited to. It will tell you if a particular medical treatment is right for you.

As you are going about your day, you can get to know your intuition by trying to hear what it is guiding you to do. You can play with it as though it were a game. For example, when you wake up, you can listen to your intuition to decide whether you will need to take a sweater in case it gets chilly outside later on. Then at lunch, ask your intuition what would be the best choice on the menu to make your body feel energized. And when you get home from work, ask your intuition if you should go to the health club and work out or if you need to stay home and rest.

As you are listening for your intuitive messages, be aware of your intellect. Does your intellect try to override your intuition's guidance? For example, regarding taking a sweater, your intuition may say, *Yes, take a sweater*, but your intellect may say, *Oh, I don't need to take a sweater. I watched the weather forecast on the news last night, and the weather will be warm. I shouldn't worry so much about getting cold*. If your intuition tells you that you should stay home and rest after work, does your intellect try to talk you into working out instead? It may say, *Even though my body is exhausted, I need to lose weight so I had better work out. I have been looking really fat and ugly lately, and I'll only lose weight if I go to the health club*.

Watch for any emotions you feel. Are you annoyed that your intuition tells you to skip dessert after lunch? Do you let your anger flow? Allow yourself to feel the emotions triggered by your intuitive messages.

As you are working on healing yourself, let your intuition be the driver, let your intellect be the GPS, and let your emotions be the fuel. With your intuition driving and your intellect and emotions working in a healthy way, you will be able to move through the unknown neighborhoods of life in an efficient way. You will find that while you may still have some painful lessons to learn, the flow of your life will be much smoother and you won't have to spend so much time on unneeded detours. And when you come to the pleasant parts of the journey, you will be able to enjoy them more fully.

▶EXERCISE: *Start trying to identify your intuition. How does it speak to you? Does it speak with a voice? with a physical sensation? in some other way?*

Look back at situations in your life in which you recognized your intuitive messages. Were there times when someone doubted what your intuition told you, so you decided not to follow it? Were there times when your own intellect doubted your intuition so you decided not to follow it? Were there times when your intuition drew you into painful learning experiences? Were there times when you followed your intuition and you had a happy outcome? Do not judge yourself for the choices you made in the past, but use this exercise to get to know your intuition so you will be able to follow it in the future.

▶EXERCISE: *Pay attention to unhealthy intellectual messages that have limited you from following your intuition. Are there messages that tell you that following your intuition is silly or your intuition isn't real? Work with these intellectual messages the way you would work with other unhealthy intellectual messages: step back, see the situations from a different perspective, and find healthy replacement messages.*

▶EXERCISE: *Listen to what your intuition is telling you about your health. What would be the healthiest diet for you? How much rest do you need? What is the right type and amount of exercise for you? What are other specific needs your body has? Pay attention to your intuitive input on a day-by-day basis. You may need different amounts of rest and different foods on some days compared to others. When your intuition tells you what your body needs, use your intellect to figure out how to meet those needs. Feel the emotions triggered by your intuitive messages, and let them fuel your energy system.*

▶ *EXERCISE: As you go about your day, pay attention to what your intuition is telling you. What does it tell you about the different people you come in contact with? What does it tell you about the different situations you are involved in? Does it tell you to change things in your life? If it does, use your intellect to figure out how you will make those changes, and feel the emotions that are triggered as you work on making those changes.*

7 Dramas

An important area of your life to work on when you are bringing your energy flow into balance is your dramas. Your dramas are all the relationships and situations in your life that trigger your emotions or cause your intellect to become hyperactive. If a person says something that makes you angry, you are in a drama with him or her. If a person does something that makes you start analyzing and judging the situation, you are in a drama with him or her. Some dramas are joyful and some are painful. The important point is that they aren't neutral, easy situations we simply breeze through. Instead, they are the situations we laugh, cry, and obsess about and lose sleep over.

Dramas can involve another person. For example, you may have a drama in the form of a conflict with your spouse. You may feel that your spouse is not doing enough work around the house, and this may make you furious. You might obsess about the fact that he always promises to do chores but then doesn't follow through. You may talk to him repeatedly and try to get him to change in an attempt to resolve the conflict.

Dramas can involve a stranger. For example, you may have a close call with an inattentive driver on the freeway. You may be furious, and you may spend the rest of the day remembering the details of what the driver did, but there is nothing you can say or do to the driver to let him know how you feel about him. The drama is alive for you as long as you are thinking about that other person.

Some dramas occur between you and an institution or a large corporation. For example, your health insurance company may change your benefits, and you may not be able to keep getting a treatment that had been approved in the past. There may not be one specific person who is responsible for the drama; instead, it involves the company as a whole. You may be angry and find yourself thinking about what a terrible insurance company you have. As long as you are thinking about the company, you are in a drama with it.

Dramas can also involve situations in which you are working on a project or a goal by yourself and there is no one else involved in the drama with you. For example, if you are creating a piece of art or trying to learn how to play a new sport, you can get caught up in the drama of your project. You may have days of frustration alternating with days of joy. You may find yourself planning and worrying about how things will turn out.

While some dramas bring us joy and fulfillment, we seem to focus more intensely on the ones that bring us pain, anger, and fear. All dramas are powerful learning experiences, and the painful ones are especially educational. They teach us important things about ourselves. Dramas are important not only because of what they teach us but also because we put many of our energy units every day into them. To heal yourself, you will need to heal your dramas and take back as many energy units from them as possible.

One common lesson that comes to us through our dramas involves emotions. Remember that the process of feeling our emotions is a natural, healthy body function. But because most of us are taught to block our emotions, our bodies frequently need to get creative to find a way to let them flow. We learn from our tribes that while some situations are not acceptable triggers for our emotions, others are. We regularly use our relationships with the people closest to us as acceptable emotional triggers. For example, you may have had a tough day at work and have some anger to feel, but you may not be allowing yourself to feel it. You are holding the lid on the emotional organ tightly closed, but the emotions are building up.

When you get home from work, your husband may say something to annoy you. His comment may be just the trigger you need to open the lid on your emotional organ and allow your anger to spew out. You may start an argument with him. Later on, you will probably regret your behavior because you realize that what he said wasn't as bad as you had thought. When you step back and review the situation, you will see how the drama wasn't actually about your husband at all. It was really about you and how you needed to create the drama in order to feel your emotions.

Dramas aren't just about emotions. They also act as mirrors to show us unhealthy intellectual messages that are deeply entrenched in our intellects and that we may not realize are there. For example, your tribe may have taught you the message that people should only need six hours of sleep, but you may actually need eight hours or you feel awful the next day. You may not realize that you have an unhealthy approach to sleep until it comes to light in a continuing drama in which you have arguments with your spouse in the mornings because you are tired and cranky.

Dramas also teach us how to make changes in our lives. You may need to learn about how to take better care of yourself. Maybe your job is draining your energy. It might be hard for you to face the fact that this is the wrong job for you. Or maybe the problem is that you don't put limits on how much energy you will put into your job. You may find yourself in a drama where you feel abused by your employer. As you work through the drama, you realize it is teaching you that you need to either change jobs or change the way you deal with the responsibilities of your job. The fact that your employer treats you poorly is less of an issue than your inner conflict over the job.

When we deal with dramas, most of us learn to focus outside ourselves, looking at the details of the situation and trying to figure out how to fix it. We analyze the other people involved and try to figure out why they did what they did. You may ask yourself, *What were they thinking? How could they do such a terrible thing to me?* You may review the details of the situation and ask yourself what you could have done differently: *Should I have said something else or changed myself in some way to make them happy?* Or you may think that if you could talk to the other people involved and get them to change, things would get better.

One problem with focusing on the other people in the drama is that you may not be able to change them. They may have different ideas than you do about how to resolve the issue. When you ask them to change for you, they may simply say no. Or they may agree to change, but over time you may notice that they don't follow through with their promises. When you try to change yourself to resolve the issue, you may find that you may not be able to change yourself enough to make them happy. Or you may find that changing yourself is unhealthy for you.

Another problem with focusing on the other people in the drama is that you may miss out on the lesson that it has to teach you. Unfortunately, dramas tend to repeat themselves over and over again until you finally learn the lesson they have to teach you. You may repeat the drama by having the same conflict with the same person, or your conflicts may have the same theme but happen with different people. Either way, the dramas will continue until you finally learn the lessons they have to teach you.

Your goal will be to stop the cycle of endless dramas. You will want to get beyond the surface details of the situations in your dramas so you can deal with the deeper issues that are there. You will want to learn whatever you need to from every drama you find yourself involved in, no matter how big or small it is. A seemingly minor drama with an annoying neighbor is as important as a serious conflict with your child. They both have something to teach you about yourself.

As you are working on changing your approach to your dramas, the first step is to focus on yourself, putting all your energy into recognizing your role in your dramas. Only when you are closely observing yourself can you change the way you deal with them. A good way to get started with this is to visualize your whole life as a big drama with you in the starring role. Imagine that you are a movie or television star. See yourself starring in your own movie, reality show, or soap opera. You are the star in your show, and the people in your life are the supporting actors.

This drama is focusing on you in every scene. Your spouse, children, friends, and coworkers are all secondary in this show. No one can ever take the spotlight away from you. When someone is in a scene with you, he or she is only there as a supporting actor. Although it would be tempting to sometimes give up your responsibility for your thoughts and actions in a scene, in this show everything is about you and only you. The camera is always focused on you; it zooms in on your face and sees your emotions, it records every thought you have, and it follows your every action.

Every single scene in your drama is all about you, and there are no exceptions to this rule, even if the action appears to be totally about someone else. For example, you may need to bring your father to the emergency room while he is having a heart attack. Although he is temporarily the center of the action in the emergency room and it would seem that he is the star of this scene, in reality you are still the star of the show.

You may not be the star of the physical action in the hospital, but you can quietly pay attention to your own part in the drama. You can visualize the scene unfolding with the doctors and nurses surrounding your father. But you also see yourself, the star of the show, standing off to the side looking anxious or upset. You can hear the thoughts going through your head. Every scene is about you. It is about your thoughts and your emotions, even when other people are involved in the action.

The purpose of this new perspective is not for you to become a selfish drama queen or king. Instead, the purpose is for you to learn to pay as close attention to yourself as possible. You will want to focus on what you think and say and how you act toward other people. You will want to notice habits you have as you live out your dramas. For example, you may notice that you have a tendency to try to manipulate people into giving you what you want. Or you may see how you are always focused on what everyone else needs and tend to ignore what you need. There are many things you may notice about yourself. Some things you may like and some may be uncomfortable to acknowledge.

Try not to judge what you see when you watch yourself in your drama. If you judge yourself, you may limit yourself from facing some of the more important lessons there are for you to learn. So remind yourself of the importance of nonjudgment, and be as open and honest with yourself as you can be.

An important thing to recognize as you watch yourself in your drama is that all the people in your life are living their own dramas as well. They are starring in their own reality shows at the same time you are starring in yours. You play a supporting role in their dramas just as they play supporting roles in yours. Your spouse has his own show to star in, and when he leaves you to go to work and do his daily activities, he has an entirely different supporting cast involved in his life than you do. Even your children have their own dramas to act out. When they are at school, they have their own cast of supporting actors, including their teachers and the other children in their classes.

Just as you are one hundred percent responsible for the way you deal with the dramas in your life, everyone else is responsible for the way they handle their own dramas. When you are worrying about the people in your life, you can remind yourself that they have the right to live out their own dramas. Of course you are going to be there for them when you can, but you can only go so far. This concept is especially important for parents. When your children are young, you are the main supporting actor in their dramas, but eventually they are going to grow up and will need to learn how to work through their dramas on their own. It can be hard to stand by and give them the independence to make their own decisions and learn from their own mistakes. But if you don't, you will be standing in the way of their personal growth.

Another situation in which it is important to remember that everyone has the right and the responsibility to live out their own dramas is when you do your drama work but the people around you don't want you to change. They may be happy with the way things have always been, and they may try to prevent you from doing your inner work so you don't rock the boat. Maybe your changes will require them to look at themselves more closely in ways they would prefer to avoid. You never want to act in a way that deliberately hurts another person, but sometimes you will bring lessons to them as you are doing your work to heal yourself. Remember that there may be a lesson for them to learn from the drama, and if you avoid doing your work in an attempt to protect them, you may be preventing them from going forward with their personal growth.

Your goal now is to focus on your drama and no one else's. Every morning when you wake up, you can imagine the television cameras turning on, following you around, and recording everything that you do. In your mind you can step back and watch the scenes as they unfold. No one else may be watching this show, and they won't know everything you are thinking or feeling, but the important thing is that you do. You want to be as fully aware as possible as you act out your life every day. You want to be focusing as intensely on yourself as you would if you were the director of the movie, viewing the action directly through the camera lens.

As you are looking at your life with this new viewpoint, you want to start seeing that every situation in your life is really an opportunity to get to know yourself better. Instead of a conflict being about what another person has done to you, you want to start seeing it as being one hundred percent about you, a lesson for you to learn from and grow from. If you find your intellect obsessing about a situation and trying to figure it out, there is something for you to learn from it. If a situation triggers a strong emotion, there is something for you to learn from it. As you work with your dramas from this point of view, you will be able to get to the root of why they are a problem for you, and then you will be able to heal them. As you heal your dramas you will be able to reallocate the energy units you have been spending on them into healthier activities.

▶*EXERCISE: Spend a few days focusing closely on yourself as the star of your own movie, reality show, or soap opera. Give the show a name, for example, "The Stephanie Show." Have some fun with it, and imagine that you are watching yourself as you are going through your daily activities. Observe yourself during your interactions with other people. See your body language as you respond to other people. Listen to the internal monologue running through your head. See the emotions on your face. See your actions as you deal with different situations. Try not to judge yourself. Just observe.*

▶*EXERCISE: Look at the people in your life, and see how they all are starring in their own dramas. Identify the supporting actors and themes in their dramas. Recognize that you need to allow them to live out their own dramas while you are living out yours.*

The Drama Within the Drama

Now that you are focusing on yourself as the star of your drama, you will want to identify situations and dramas within the drama that are there to teach you something. You will want to identify all situations, no matter how big or small. It doesn't matter if it is a little drama over your spouse not picking up his dirty clothes or if it is a big drama over your boss firing you. You will want to work on every situation that bothers you, no matter how important it appears to be. Ordinarily culture tells us to ignore the small stuff and address only the big issues. We aren't supposed to get worked up over little things because they are supposed to be inconsequential. We are taught, *Don't cry over spilt milk*. But in reality, every situation that triggers our thoughts or emotions is important. You will find that there are a lot of lessons to be learned from the small dramas. And you will find that if you learn your lessons from the small dramas, you will be able to more easily work through the big ones.

Once you have identified a drama you need to deal with, you will want to step back and start to do your work. This work will involve you and only you. It will not involve the other people in the drama. Don't say anything to them, and don't do anything to fix the situation yet. The action steps you need to take will come later. Instead, step back and focus on yourself and do your inner work first.

The only exceptions to this rule of doing your own inner work first are situations in which you or another person is in immediate danger or when you have to take care of something, such as going to a special event or taking care of your children's needs. In those cases you should do what you need to do to take care of things first. You can go back later and review the situation and learn what you need to once things have been taken care of.

As you are focusing on doing your inner work, you will want to step back and look at the drama through the director's camera lens, watching yourself as closely as you can. Most of the work you need to do is going to be done by yourself, with yourself. Only when you have done your work and learned what you need to learn should you try to take action. This way your action will come not from a place of projected emotion or judgment, but from a place of inner knowing of what will be the most beneficial action for the situation.

Start your work by trying to feel your emotions. Allow them to flow as freely as possible. It is always the most beneficial thing to feel the emotions triggered by your dramas while you are going through the dramas. This is the opposite of what we are usually taught. Usually people get taught to use their intellects to analyze the details of a drama and to judge themselves and the other people involved. They are taught to try to figure out how they can change themselves or the other people involved in the drama. But the approach of using excessive intellectual activity to try to control the situation doesn't help you get to the root of the problem. You may find a solution for this specific drama, but you may not have learned what you need to. This could lead to your having to repeat the same drama over and over again.

So instead of thinking too much about the drama, you should step off the intellectual treadmill and feel the emotions that are triggered by the situation. For example, if your boss criticized your work this morning, notice your response. You may catch yourself obsessing all day and analyzing the reasons for the criticism. As you step back and observe yourself, you can see that you are on the intellectual treadmill. Obviously this situation is a drama with something to teach you because you are thinking so much about it. Recognize that your intellect has been triggered, and instead of getting stuck on the intellectual treadmill, let yourself feel your emotions. Maybe you are angry or hurt. Or maybe you are feeling fear about losing your job. Feel your emotions as deeply as you can.

Although this drama is all about you and what you need to learn about yourself, it is natural in the beginning to focus your attention on the other people involved. If you need to visualize their faces to bring out your anger or sadness, do it. Just remember, in the back of your mind, that although this conflict may seem to be about both you and the other people involved, your goal is to ultimately focus only on yourself and your role in it. As important as the other people seem to be, at this point focusing on how to fix them or change them won't help you. Recognize that you are the star of your drama and they are just your costars in this scene, acting as triggers for your emotions and helping you learn something. Changing your perspective this way can be difficult, but do your best to always keep the camera lens focused on yourself.

Remember that you cannot project your emotions onto the other people involved in the drama. You can't yell at them or cry to them or tell them how they hurt you. You can't waste your energy trying to talk to them or reason with them or get them to see your side of the conflict. You will deal with them later. Right now your only job is to feel your emotions. You need to let yourself feel as strongly about the situation as you need to, no matter how silly your intellect judges your emotions to be.

No matter how small the situation may seem, your emotional response can't be judged. If the drama is over something that appears small, such as your annoyance with your son for spilling his breakfast on the floor, you still need to let yourself feel your emotions. Don't tell yourself, *This isn't a big deal; it wasn't his fault for spilling; I'll just let it go*. Instead, think, *Every drama, big or small, needs to be dealt with. It may not be his fault for spilling, but I'm still mad that I have to clean it up*. Let yourself feel the emotions triggered by the situation for as long as you need to. For a small spill you may be angry for only a few minutes. For bigger dramas you may feel an emotion for many hours at a time. It may take days or weeks or months of intense emotional work. The amount of time it takes cannot be judged. It may not make sense why you are feeling such deep emotions over a relatively small drama, but don't waste your energy trying to figure it out.

There are a number of reasons for doing your emotion work by yourself without involving other people. One reason is that we frequently create dramas to give ourselves a culturally sanctioned reason to feel our emotions. Remember that there is a lot of judgment and shame surrounding emotions. If you wake up feeling cranky one morning, you may have trouble spontaneously letting your anger flow because the judgments you've internalized say that anger is bad. You may have learned that the only way you can feel anger is if someone else triggers it in you. So on those cranky days, you may find yourself looking around defensively, just waiting for someone to do something to make you mad. It's as though that person has to give you permission to feel your anger. This will tempt you to blame that person for your anger when it actually has nothing to do with him or her.

Another reason for doing your emotion work on your own is that you may find times when your emotions are very intense. This is especially common when people first start feeling their emotions this new way. Some days you may feel somewhat out of control as your emotions flood out of you. Your body can be so relieved to release the pent-up emotions that it can send wave after wave of them through you. If a drama comes up and triggers them, it can be tempting to become overly dramatic and project them onto the other people involved in the drama. You don't want to hurt those other people by projecting your emotions onto them. It's much better to do your emotion work on your own and deal with the other people later.

You will also want to do your emotion work before you deal with the details of a drama so your emotions don't get in the way of resolving the drama. For example, if your husband promised to clean the garage but didn't do it and you are angry, you will be tempted to talk to him with an angry and accusatory voice. He will probably respond by getting defensive and projecting anger back at you. This will escalate the drama. When you are communicating this way, you won't be able to resolve the issue. It is much healthier to do your emotion work on your own and then come to the table and discuss the issue when you are feeling less emotional. You will often find that the other person in the conflict will respond to you in a different way, and you will get more accomplished when you are not projecting your emotions.

One last reason to feel your emotions immediately during a drama is because if you don't let yourself feel them, you will end up holding them in your body, in your emotional basement. The emotional basement holds all the emotions from your past that you were taught not to feel. Every time you had a drama and didn't allow your emotions to flow, you put those emotions into a room in the emotional basement. Now that you have started to work on clearing out all the pent-up emotions from your past, the last thing you will want to do is fill the basement up again.

With some dramas the main lesson is simply to feel emotions.

You will know this is the case if, with time, your emotions become less intense and the drama stops upsetting you. Maybe you got a prank phone call that made you very angry. After breathing the anger through your emotional organ for ten minutes, you find that you are ready to let it go and you don't care about it anymore. You see that the drama was just a situation to trigger some anger, and now it's over.

But sometimes there is more to learn from a drama than that you need to feel your emotions. You may find that the situation continues to bother you even after you have felt your emotions. Or maybe you notice that you have the same conflict over and over again and the process of feeling your emotions isn't enough to resolve it for good. If you find yourself being unable to let go of a drama after you have been feeling your emotions, you will want to focus also on what the drama has to teach you about your intellect.

Your dramas are valuable in showing you the unhealthy intellectual messages you have internalized, especially the messages that are more subtle and difficult to recognize. Many intellectual messages we learn from our tribes can be so deeply entrenched that we can have trouble seeing them. You can use your dramas to help you identify the messages that are especially problematic for you.

To identify the unhealthy messages that a drama is showing you, start by asking yourself what it is that the other person in the drama is doing to you or what quality in the other person bothers you so much. If the drama involves you alone, ask yourself what bothers you so much about the situation.

Often the answer is that you feel you are being hurt by the other person in the conflict or they aren't being respectful of you. For example, if you are a parent in a drama with children who never do their chores, you may feel hurt by your children. When they don't do their chores, you end up staying up late at night doing the work they were supposed to do. You may realize that your children don't care that you have to stay up late to do their chores. With their actions, your children are telling you they don't care about your needs and don't respect you.

When you are working on this step of the process, don't judge the situation or try to explain away what the other person is doing. It may be hard to look at your sweet, beloved children and think that your children don't care about or respect you. If you are having a conflict with a child, a person who is more vulnerable than you, or someone who cares about you, still be honest with yourself and ask what they are doing to you, even if they don't necessarily realize they are hurting or using you. Remember that this lesson is for you alone and it is not something you need to discuss with anyone else. You won't be hurting anyone else's feelings by acknowledging what you think the other person in the drama is doing to you. And you may find that sometimes, what you think they are doing is more imagined by you rather than being something they are actually doing.

In addition to looking at what the other person in the drama is doing to you, explore any behaviors or qualities that bother you in that other person. For example, when you look at the drama with your children who don't do their chores, the problem may not just be that they are disrespectful of you. It may also be that you are bothered because they don't take responsibility for themselves or that they are lazy.

For every type of drama, you will want to apply this step of looking at what the other person is doing to you or what quality in him or her bothers you. Do this with dramas involving institutions and groups of people too. Ask yourself what the group as a whole is doing to you or what quality you find bothersome about the group. For example, if your city makes you give up your land because of an issue over eminent domain, you may feel that the city government is victimizing you. You may be bothered by the government's lack of respect for the individuals it is supposed to support.

If your drama seems to involve you alone, ask yourself what the situation is doing to you. For example, if you are an artist working on a painting that isn't going well, ask yourself what bothers you about this situation. Does the situation seem to hold you hostage, blocking you from finding your creative spark? Does the situation limit you because you have time or financial constraints that stop you from accomplishing what you know you have the potential to accomplish? Try to identify what specific things in the situation are limiting your forward movement.

Each drama will have its own set of things that will bother you. Some dramas will have one issue for you to work with, but some dramas will have many. Sometimes you will know immediately what it is in the drama that bothers you. But in other situations it will take time to figure out. You need to give yourself time to figure out exactly what is bothering you. Don't rush this step. Don't lie to yourself and say that the other person didn't really mean to hurt you. You need to be as clear as possible to yourself about what you think is happening to you in the situation. The more detailed and honest you are with this step, the more you will learn about yourself.

Once you have figured out what the other person in the situation has done to you or what quality in them bothers you, you will want to move on to the next step. This step takes much introspection, and it can be the most difficult aspect of healing your dramas. Now you will want to pick up the proverbial mirror and use it to reflect the external details of the situation back onto yourself. You will use it to see that everything the other person is doing to you, you are also actually doing to yourself. Every quality that bothers you in that other person is also a quality that you possess. For example, if you feel that someone is hurting you, look for a place in your life where you are hurting yourself or someone else. If you feel that someone is disrespectful of you, look for a place in your life where you are disrespectful of yourself or someone else. If you don't like someone because they have the quality of being critical and they criticize you, there is a part of you that is also critical of yourself or others.

These qualities that are being mirrored for you may involve this particular drama or they may exhibit themselves in other situations. If you are the parent who is upset because your children don't want to take responsibility for their chores, see how in some area of your life you also aren't taking responsibility for something. It may be in this drama over your children's chores, or it may be that you aren't taking responsibility in another part of your life.

In this situation with your children, you may realize that you aren't taking responsibility for teaching them the lessons about being self-reliant and how to be respectful and responsible. You may be very busy, and you may have simply gotten in the habit of doing their work for them. In the short run, it may have seemed easier to do their work for them rather than take the time to figure out how to teach them how to take responsibility for themselves.

Or maybe you realize that the problem is that you have a tendency to not take responsibility for yourself in other situations. Maybe you have a tendency to just go along with what other people want, even when what they want hurts you. You may have learned when you were young that it is more important to make other people happy than it is to take care of yourself. The end result of this is you are not taking responsibility for yourself and you are not getting what you need.

You will also want to use the mirror to help you understand yourself better in dramas where some characteristic or quality in someone else bothers you. After you have identified what it is that bothers you about them, ask yourself where you possess that quality inside of yourself. For example, someone in your life may be very controlling. They may annoy you because they try to control you. And they may be annoying because they are very self-controlled and uptight. Now you want to look at yourself and see where you have a tendency to be controlling. Maybe you try to control other people. Or maybe you try to control yourself in order to fit into your tribes and make other people happy.

If you have a drama with an institution or a tribe, ask yourself what quality possessed by the tribe or what activity being done by the tribe bothers you. Then look at yourself to see how you possess that quality or where you do the same thing they are doing. For example, you may have a situation at work in which you feel your company doesn't appreciate the way you do your job. You may feel your supervisors want you to do the job in a way that you consider to be inadequate. Maybe they want you to cut corners or do things that you think are unethical.

As you look in the mirror, you may see that your company is showing you the part of yourself that is willing to be unethical. As long as you continue to work for this company, you aren't appreciating yourself because you are allowing the quality of your work to be compromised. Maybe you realize that as long as you continue to stay in this situation, you aren't living up to your full potential.

You will want to apply the mirror concept to situations in which you are having a drama with yourself over something that you are trying to create. For example, if you are an artist and you feel blocked and you can't move forward, you may be focused on the external situation and think that you are being blocked by your lack of the right tools or resources. Pay attention to what you think the situation is doing to limit you. Then pick up the mirror and ask yourself where you are limiting yourself. Are you blocked because there is something inside you that is blocked? Is there some inner work you need to do to allow your energy to flow more fully? Maybe you are blocked creatively because you aren't allowing yourself to hear your intuition. Maybe you need to rest and get a different perspective.

Often you will find that the issues your dramas mirror for you are connected to unhealthy intellectual messages you believe in. The unhealthy intellectual messages you internalize from your tribes may be so deeply ingrained that it can be hard to recognize them. Your dramas are a very powerful source for helping you identify those deeper messages.

For example, you may be in a drama with someone who is critical of you. You may have previously thought the problem was totally about that other person, but as you do your work with the mirror, you can see that the other person is, more importantly, showing you a part of yourself that is critical. Maybe you are critical of someone else, but you may also be critical of yourself. You may have internalized a message telling you that you are not good enough the way you are. This current drama with the critical person is here to help you recognize that message. So while on the surface the drama seems to be all about the problem with that critical person, the real drama is between you and the intellectual message that says you are not good enough.

It is important to remember that only the intellectual messages we truly believe will be mirrored by another person in a drama. If you have learned to judge yourself harshly, you will find yourself getting upset about a drama in which someone judges or criticizes you. But if you haven't internalized the message that you should judge yourself harshly, when someone criticizes you, the judgment will just flow off you like water flows off a duck's back. You can assume that if a drama is bothering you and you can't let it go, there is an unhealthy intellectual message at the root of it for you.

Once you have recognized an unhealthy intellectual message being mirrored for you, deal with it the same way you would handle any other unhealthy intellectual message. Do the exercises for calming the intellect. Step back and observe the situation from a different perspective. Find nonjudgmental, regenerative replacement messages.

There is one type of drama that may require a slightly different approach than the approach discussed here. If you have a drama in which you feel victimized by another person or situation, simply trying to pick up the mirror to deal with your victimization may not be very helpful. You may only end up feeling trapped and alone. I'll discuss how to deal with victimization later in this book.

When you feel that you have learned what you need to learn from a drama, the last thing to do is to take action. By now you have done your work with your emotions and your intellect. You have come to understand the lessons that the drama has to teach you. Now you will want to move forward and take any actions that are needed to bring the details in your external life into alignment with your new understanding of your inner self.

The action that you need to make depends on the individual drama. Usually you have a few basic choices about how to proceed. If you realize that the drama's purpose was mostly to trigger an emotion, once you have felt the emotion you will find yourself letting go of the drama. For example, if you were really angry when another driver cut you off and you have felt all the anger, you will naturally let it go and move on.

If you find that you have hurt another person because you have projected your emotions onto him or her, you need to apologize. You also need to recognize when you are falling into a similar pattern in the future so you can prevent it from happening again. This is why it is so important to learn how to feel your emotions in a healthy way. The more comfortable you get with feeling your emotions, the fewer dramas you will create with them.

If you realize that a drama requires you to make a significant change in your life, you need to put your energy toward making the change. You can use your intuition to help you decide what action to take. For example, if you are unhappy with your job, you may realize that you need to change careers. You may need to seek support from family or friends, and it may take time for you to figure out how to make the change. You don't necessarily need to rush the change. Sometimes you will need to stop and rest and wait for a while. You will know what to do when the time is right.

If you have a drama that involves a conflict with another person, you may need to work with that other person to resolve the conflict. For example, if you and your wife have a conflict over how to discipline your teenager, you need to come to an agreement about how to approach the issue; you know that a change is needed, so decide what to do next.

In this scenario, after you have done your work with your emotions and your intellect, sit down and figure out exactly what you need from your spouse. Use your intuition to help you know what you need, then discuss it with her. You want this discussion to be as unemotional and drama-free as possible. You may find that because you have stepped back and taken yourself out of the drama, you will be able to communicate more effectively with her. And she may respond to you differently than she had in the past. She may now recognize your new sense of inner resolve, and you may find that even though you are dealing with the same old conflict, she may be more willing to work with you than she had been before.

The hard part in any drama comes if the other person involved isn't willing to work with you to resolve it. If that is the case, you have to accept that the other person isn't willing to change. Usually you then have two options: either allow things to stay the way they are or do what you need to do to take care of yourself. Do the drama steps again. Feel your emotions, do your intellect work, and listen to your intuitive guidance to know what action step to take.

It can be hard to contemplate doing something that the other person involved in the conflict doesn't want you to do. She may pressure you to keep things the way they are. She may like things this way, and she may want to avoid working on her own lessons in the drama. If this is the case, step back and observe the situation from her perspective. Recognize that she also has her own dramas to experience. She is starring in her own television show, and she has her own life lessons to learn.

Just as other people act as mirrors to teach you what you need to know about yourself, you also act as a mirror to teach them what they need to know about themselves. In an ideal world, we all would take one hundred percent responsibility for ourselves and would work on learning the lessons our dramas have to teach us. But in reality this is not so easy. It is common for people to try to avoid learning their life lessons. They avoid feeling the emotions triggered by their dramas, and they have a difficult time taking their focus off the outside world and putting it onto themselves.

While it can be hard to take action steps that will create dramas for other people, you need to remember that it is not your right to judge what they need to learn. If your work on a drama takes you in a direction that causes some upheaval in other people's lives, maybe they also have something to learn from the situation. Don't stop your own personal growth with the excuse that you want to protect them from feeling emotions or learning more about themselves.

If you trigger a drama that other people need to grow from, you may actually be doing them a favor by helping them see parts of themselves that need healing. So take the action that your intuition guides you to take; do what is best for yourself in the situation. You will find that when you act in this responsible way, having done your inner work first and listening to your intuition for guidance, what is most beneficial for you will be most beneficial for everyone involved.

An important thing to remember as you work with your dramas is that this is a process. Your goal isn't to decide what action to take by tomorrow or next week. You should take as much time as you need to work with the emotions and the intellectual messages triggered by a drama. See the process of working through your dramas as a tool for helping you get to know yourself better. With some dramas you may take months to learn all the lessons you need to learn. By approaching your dramas this way, you will find that when you finally take action, there will be a sense of peace in it.

You can also use this approach for working through past dramas that you haven't resolved yet. You can work through a drama that occurred last week, last month, or even twenty years ago. Working through your past dramas can help you clean out your emotional basement. It can also help you learn lessons about unhealthy intellectual messages you are holding on to. We tend to repeat dramas over and over again until we learn the lessons that they are trying to teach us. The people involved and the details may change, but the themes will be consistent until we have finally learned the lesson. Sometimes it is easier to look back and learn a lesson from a past drama than it is to see a lesson in a current situation.

You will know that a past drama is still an issue for you if you still get upset every time you think about it. Or maybe you find your intellect judging the situation and getting on the intellectual treadmill and obsessing over it. Or maybe you find yourself trying to not think about it at all.

Maybe you have unresolved grief over someone's death, or maybe you still feel betrayed by a friend in a situation that happened years ago. Or maybe you feel shame over something you did to someone else. Whatever the details of the drama are, be aware that if you haven't been able to come to a sense of peace over it, there is still work to be done. Of course if something very traumatic happened in the past, you may always feel emotions connected to it. But if you find the memory of the situation continually coming back to haunt you and you find yourself stewing over it or working hard to forget it, you had better work through it so you can finally lay it to rest.

You may have talked about a past drama with a friend, family member, or psychologist, and you may think that you've worked through the drama; you've forgiven the other person, and it isn't a problem for you anymore. But be aware that talking about a situation is not the same as feeling your emotions about the situation. Your intellect may have come to a place where it can explain the situation in a way that it is comfortable with, but if you haven't felt the emotions, the drama will still have a hold on you.

You may also look back at a drama and say that you have done the action steps needed to resolve it, so you may assume you have let it go. But if you haven't felt the emotions triggered by the drama and haven't learned all that the drama was mirroring for you, it will continue taking your energy. You will know this is happening if you resolve one drama only to find yourself experiencing a similar drama later on.

An example of this is what can happen with abuse victims. People who have been abused will often leave one abusive situation only to get involved in another. They may have taken action and gotten out of the first relationship, but if they didn't allow themselves to feel all the emotions associated with the abuse, they couldn't really process the drama fully. And if they didn't identify the unhealthy intellectual messages the abuser was mirroring for them, they will still believe those messages and will continue to be vulnerable to being abused again.

When you recognize a past drama you need to work on, you can approach it the same way you approach current dramas. Step back and witness yourself in the drama. Let the situation trigger your emotions, and let yourself feel them for as long as you need to. Also do the work to identify the unhealthy intellectual messages the situation was mirroring for you. Finally, take action if something needs to be done. But frequently there won't be anything more to do. Often the point of working through past dramas is more about cleaning out your emotional basement and learning lessons about yourself than actually changing the situation.

You will find that working through your dramas will help your energy flow. Allowing your emotions to flow will fuel your energy system. Discovering your unhealthy intellectual messages and calming them will free up the energy units they had been using. Taking action and changing unhealthy situations will pull your energy away from those situations and bring it back into your own body. As you heal your dramas you will also heal yourself.

▶ *EXERCISE: Pay attention to a drama in your life and apply the first step to working through it: witness yourself in the drama, and step back and let your emotions be triggered by the drama. Don't discuss the drama or try to resolve the situation with the other people involved; instead, give yourself time to work through it on your own. Let yourself feel your emotions as deeply and as long as you need to, and don't judge them.*

You may find that after feeling your emotions, the drama is resolved and the lesson in it was for you to simply feel emotions. If you find that you drew someone into your drama by projecting your emotions onto them, apologize to them.

If you realize there is something more to learn from the drama, go to the next step and ask yourself, What did the other people in the situation do to bother me? *or* What quality in those other people is upsetting me? *If the situation is about you alone, ask yourself,* What has the situation itself done to upset me?

Once you have a very specific understanding of what bothers you about those other people or the situation, pick up the proverbial mirror and see that whatever is being done to you is the exact same thing you are doing to yourself or someone else. And if there is a quality in the other person in the drama that is bothering you, use the mirror to see where that quality exists inside yourself.

If you find that the drama has helped you recognize an unhealthy intellectual message you believe in, do the work needed to let go of that message.

Finally, if you find that a change is needed, make an action plan to change the situation. Use your intuition to help you choose what action to take. Remember that if your drama involves other people and you need to talk with them about resolving the drama, don't project your emotions onto them, and remember that your job is to work on your part of the drama, not theirs. If the drama brings up issues or emotions for them, acknowledge their right and responsibility to do their own drama work, but don't limit your forward growth so they can avoid doing their own work.

▶EXERCISE: *Observe other people's dramas as a way to appreciate the concept of dramas more clearly. Observe dramas you read about in the newspaper and books. Watch for dramas on television and in movies. Observe dramas that your friends and family experience. Apply the steps above and imagine yourself in the other people's dramas. Imagine the emotions, the intellectual lessons, and the potential action steps to be taken. This exercise may be able to help you work through your own dramas more easily. But don't use this exercise as a reason to become a busybody. Don't give other people advice on how to deal with their dramas unless they ask you for it.*

▶ *EXERCISE: Watch for dramas from your past that you still haven't come to peace with. If you find yourself repeatedly thinking about or avoiding the memories of a past drama, or if you realize you still have emotions in your emotional basement connected to an old drama, work through it the same way you would deal with a current drama. The main difference may be that with old dramas you don't have the same options for action steps that you do with current ones.*

8 Life Lessons and Archetypes

While it would be nice for life to always be full of fun and joy, in reality we all have times of sorrow and suffering. We all have lessons to learn, and unfortunately, those lessons often bring pain. While we may wish that we could avoid the pain of life, it is impossible to expect that we will never experience painful life lessons.

An example of a painful life lesson is illness. When patients are sick and lose their ability to function normally, they can wonder, *Why did this happen to me? Why do I have to suffer like this when all the people around me seem to be so happy and healthy?* People who are sick are not the only ones who experience losses and wonder, *Why me?* We all have times in our lives when we have to deal with challenging experiences that cause us pain. When you are going through those times, you can feel isolated and alone. You can feel that no one understands you and that God has it in for you. You may ask God what you did to deserve this. You can feel a sense of victimization, as though you are trapped and have no control over your life.

We all have different life lessons we have to work through. We might not have to face these lessons every day; we might have periods in our lives that are easy and carefree. But then we might have a run of "bad luck" when nothing works out right. The details vary from person to person, but we all share the common experience of having to work through our difficult life lessons at some time during our lives.

The problem with these life lessons is that we are taught by culture —especially Western culture—that we are never supposed to have pain or times of struggle. We are taught that we are supposed to be happy, successful, rich, beautiful, and thin. We are supposed to think positive thoughts and always have smiles on our faces. We aren't supposed to complain about our misery or admit we are afraid. We are taught to create an image that helps us cover up our uncomfortable emotions and our struggles. It's as though we create a happy mask that we can put on when we need to cover up any imperfections that may be lurking deep inside us.

There is a problem with putting on the happy mask and pretending that everything is okay. When you always pretend that things are okay, the happy mask can become glued so firmly into place that it doesn't come off easily. When a painful life lesson comes along, you may not be able to communicate to the people around you about how much you are suffering. If they don't know you are suffering, they won't be able to support you, and you can feel isolated and alone.

When you are wearing the happy mask, you can also be tempted to lie to yourself about the reality of your situation. You can go into a state of denial and pretend that you don't have the problems you are having. This may cause you to make unhealthy choices that prolong your misery. For example, you may be having financial problems, and you may really need to stop spending so much money. But if your happy mask won't allow you to admit to yourself that you have a big a problem, you may continue to spend money you don't have. The longer you wait to deal with your problem, the bigger it will become.

When you don't face your problems and work through them, you can end up bringing your energy flow out of balance. As your intellect works to deny the reality of the situation, it wastes valuable energy units on its unhealthy thought patterns. And if you don't allow yourself to feel the emotions associated with the situation, you can also block your energy flow. To be healthy you need to take off the happy mask—at least with yourself—so you can work through your life lessons and heal them and bring balance to your energy flow.

There are myriad lessons we experience in life. For people born into families that are neglectful or abusive, the first big lesson starts when they are born. Neglect and abuse can have devastating consequences. When you have been abused as a child, it can affect everything that happens to you for the rest of your life. You did not choose to be born into an abusive family, but you will have to deal with the life lessons it teaches you whether you want to or not.

Another common lesson that life brings young children involves their sense of belonging in their tribes. You may not have been abused as a child, but you may have been born into a dysfunctional family and taught unhealthy messages that made you feel inadequate. You may have been the one person in your family who didn't fit in with the rest. Maybe you were very sensitive, emotionally or physically, and your family didn't appreciate your sensitivity. Maybe you were different in the way you looked or acted. Frequently when one family member is different from the others, he or she is made to feel inadequate and unacceptable.

Whether a child is neglected, abused, or just feels left out, the situation can seem completely unfair. You can feel trapped and alone. The hard thing about having problems when you are a child is that you can't just leave the situation. Unless someone from outside the family is there to come and take you away, you can't just move out on your own. You are stuck with your family until you get old enough to take care of yourself. When you are abused or neglected as a child, you have no choice but to go through your painful experience, no matter how terrible it is.

When you've had a painful childhood, you can be tempted to put it behind you and forget it ever happened. But if you don't feel the emotions associated with the trauma, you will hold the emotions and the memory of the trauma in your body, and this is unhealthy for your energy flow. When you've had a painful childhood, you can also get into the habit of holding on to unhealthy intellectual messages you were taught when you were young. These unhealthy messages can hold you in thought patterns that limit your ability to move forward and heal yourself. For example, if you were always told that you were a bad child, you may have gotten into the habit of criticizing and judging yourself. Now years later, you may still find yourself sabotaging your success or your relationships because you have internalized the message that you are a bad person who doesn't deserve to feel joy. Until you can let go of that thought pattern you will be limited by it.

Another painful life lesson comes in the form of a random trauma, such as a car accident or a rape. After you suffer the trauma, you may spend a lot of time analyzing the situation and trying to figure out what you could have done differently to change the outcome. You may think that if you had just taken a different road to work, you wouldn't have been in the car accident. Or maybe you think that if you had just skipped that party, you could have prevented the rape.

When you experience a random trauma, it is easy for your intellect to get on the thought treadmill and tell you many different stories about the situation. It may do this to try to give you a sense of control over the situation. It may also do this as a way to help you avoid feeling the deep emotions the trauma triggered in you. If you find yourself on the intellectual treadmill after a trauma, remember that to heal the memory, you need to work on both sides of the emotion/intellect balance. You need to feel your deep emotions while you are creating new, regenerative, nonjudgmental messages to replace the unhealthy ones. An example of a new message may be: *I may never fully understand why this trauma occurred, and although my intellect can't make sense of it, I am committed to letting go of the stories that my intellect is tempted to tell. I know that I am on this earth to learn lessons, and this seems to be one of the most painful ones. The pain from this lesson is a reminder that I am living the human experience to its fullest.*

Many of us find ourselves drawn into life situations that start out full of hope and joy but end up bringing us painful lessons in the form of dramas. This can happen when we get involved in relationships with other people. These relationships can be romantic or involve friends or business partners. You may marry the person of your dreams and feel intuitively that he or she is the perfect partner for you. But then after you get married, you may realize that your spouse is a drug addict. Although you love your spouse, you also have to deal with the pain of the addiction.

Or you may have been drawn into a business partnership with a person you liked and trusted. In the beginning everything may have intuitively felt right for you and you may have been very excited about the venture. But later on the partnership may have hit some big snags, and in the end the situation may have become a total disaster. Maybe your relationship with your business partner became contentious, and in the end the originally exciting experience became a painful learning experience.

As with any other painful life lesson, when you are drawn into dramas that are originally full of promise but don't turn out as you had planned, you need to feel the emotions triggered by the situation. You also need to work with the proverbial mirror to discover and let go of any unhealthy intellectual messages the situation has to show you. Only then will you be able to make new plans and move on.

▶*EXERCISE: Identify the painful life lessons that have shaped you. Common areas where people experience these life lessons are with their health, their childhoods, seemingly random painful experiences, and relationships they are drawn into.*

▶*EXERCISE: Identify your happy mask and the things you say and do when you are trying to fake that everything is okay. What situations trigger you to put it on, or is it always glued tightly in place? Do you allow yourself or anyone else to see the truth behind your happy mask?*

It is normal for people to have a happy mask that they use to protect themselves when they are feeling vulnerable. But if you find that you never take yours off, you will need to investigate why it is so tightly plastered on. Are you trying to avoid feeling painful emotions, or are you trying to avoid dealing with a painful life lesson?

▶*EXERCISE: As you identify your painful life lessons, do your work with your unhealthy intellectual messages and your emotions, so that you can redirect your energy units from those situations to the regenerative work of healing yourself.*

Archetypes
In addition to learning life lessons through our childhood experiences, random traumas, and the relationships we are drawn into, we learn powerful life lessons through the roles we play at work, in our families, and in other areas of our lives. For example, if you are a nurse, the role you play when you are at work can bring you rich rewards, but it can also bring you difficult life lessons as you try to figure out how to deal with the stress and fatigue that are frequently part of the job. The role a scientist plays can be intellectually fascinating and challenging, but it can also bring life lessons about the need to accept the mysteries in life. The role of being a writer may bring you the lesson of how to deal with self-doubt as you try to put your ideas on to paper, but it may reward you with great joy when you see your creation in print. We all live out different life roles, and these roles bring us valuable life lessons.

A word that can be used to describe these life roles is *archetype*. An archetype is a symbol. Its meaning is understood universally, across cultures and across time. Many things take on archetypal symbolism. An object, such as a cross, can be an archetypal symbol. When many people see a cross they think of divinity. Different animals have archetypal meanings as well. For example, the bull commonly represents power and aggression, and the fox represents cunning and trickery.

Archetypal symbols get their meanings from the characteristics or stories associated with them.

Life roles take on symbolic archetypal meanings. As many people experience a certain life role, they start to have certain expectations of that role. For example, throughout time many people have been fishermen. Because we have all been exposed to fishermen, either through stories or in person, we have a picture in our minds of what they do and what we should expect from them. When we say the word *fisherman*, we envision a man fishing on the water. There may be variations in the details of how each person living the archetype experiences it, but as all fishermen live out the archetype, their experiences follow a basic theme. When we refer to that archetype, everyone understands what it represents.

Other examples of archetypes include the teacher, the mother, the warrior, the activist, and the healer. When we hear the word *teacher*, we have a very specific idea of what that role entails. We all can envision a person who personifies that role. We may think of a person who we felt was a good teacher for us when we were in school, or we may picture an actor who played the role of a good teacher in a movie. We know what teachers are supposed to accomplish: they help their pupils learn new information. If teachers achieve the goals of the teacher archetype, they will feel a sense of fulfillment. If they don't accomplish their goals, they can end up judging themselves as being inadequate.

We all experience a number of archetypal roles during our lifetimes. Some archetypes involve our work and our careers. For example, the waitress, the businessperson, the carpenter, and the farmer are archetypes symbolizing different jobs and careers. Some archetypes involve our personality types. For example, the comedian, the hero, and the princess symbolize personality types. If you know someone who makes you laugh, you may say that so-and-so is such a clown. That person may not try to make a living doing comedy, but you think of him or her as a comedian anyway. Some archetypes involve our hobbies. You may be an athlete, a musician, a cook, or a gardener. You may not do these things as a job, but these archetypes may play a significant role in your life.

Some archetypes involve our relationships to the people in our families. For example, the mother, the father, the grandparent, and the son or daughter are all common familial archetypes. Different people in the family are expected to play out their archetypal roles as society has scripted them. The father has traditionally been expected to support the family financially and act as its leader, and the mother has traditionally been responsible for nurturing the family. The children have been expected to respect their elders and follow their guidance. And as people have grown older and become grandparents, they have transitioned into the wise elder role.

Some archetypes involve aspects of our inner selves. For example, your inner child is that childlike part of you that feels your emotions and likes to play. It is the part of you that tries to be good and get people's approval, and at times it can also be a bit of a devil. Your victim archetype is the part of you that comes out in times of stress, and it can make you feel that your life is not under your control and that you are trapped and alone.

The combination of archetypes is different for everyone. Some of our archetypal roles feel very natural to us, and we enjoy experiencing them. Other archetypal roles present difficult challenges for us to work with. Each archetype you experience will have a different level of importance for you. At different times in your life, one archetype may become more important than the others, depending on what is going on with you at that time.

For example, a woman may be a teacher and a mother and an activist in her lifetime. She may focus most of her energy on her teacher archetype before her children are born. Then when her children are young, her mother archetype may be her main focus. After her children leave home, she may then focus on her activist archetype and start working to make changes in her community.

We don't tend to pick our archetypal roles out of the air and think, *Oh, I think I'll experience the clown and the gossip archetypes in this life.* Instead, we are naturally drawn to certain archetypal roles that feel right for us. We may feel that some of the roles are thrown into our laps without our asking for them, but we feel driven to live them out to the best of our ability. For example, maybe you had an unplanned pregnancy and found yourself being thrown into the role of mother. You might not have felt that you were ready to be a mother, but later on you realized that although you never would have planned it, being a mother has become one of the most fulfilling experiences in your life.

Our archetypal roles have a strong effect on our energy flow. If you have an archetype you are drawn to but don't allow yourself to experience, your energy flow might become blocked and out of balance. For example, you may have always wanted to be an artist, but you might not have taken the time to get to know that part of yourself. Maybe you feel that you aren't talented enough or don't have enough time to do it. The reason you decided not to pursue your art doesn't matter. The fact is that if you ignore your artist archetype, you may be missing out on an important experience that will enhance your energy flow and your personal growth.

Our archetypes have an important impact on our energy flow while we are experiencing them. Because our archetypes are so important to us, we tend to put a lot of our energy into the work they require. If you look at where you spend your one hundred energy units every day, you will probably find yourself putting large amounts of energy into your archetypal roles. A stock trader may find that he puts ninety energy units every day into trading stocks. A surgeon may spend almost all her energy units on a given day on an especially challenging surgery.

Because of all the energy your archetypal roles require, you will want to pay close attention to the details of how you live them. You will want to be true to the archetypal roles that are important to you.

You will need to accept the challenges they offer you in order to facilitate healthy energy flow. But at the same time, you will want to recognize that you need to have balance in all areas of your life, including the work you do in your archetypal roles. It is not healthy to sacrifice your physical health or your inner peace for the sake of your archetypal roles.

You will want to work with your archetypes and make sure you are living them in a balanced way. To do this, it is important that you recognize and heal any unhealthy intellectual messages or judgments you associate with them. Because many archetypes have been around for such a long time, they tend to have a lot of outdated intellectual messages attached to them. For example, an outdated intellectual message associated with the Cinderella archetype is that she needs a Prince Charming to fulfill her wishes. The new intellectual message associated with the Cinderella archetype is that she can find fulfillment herself without having to wait for her prince to provide that for her. It is your job to recognize when you have an outdated intellectual message attached to your archetypal role, and it is your responsibility to change the message to a healthy, more regenerative one. You can then change your life to fit your new message.

We all live our own individual constellation of archetypal roles. As you observe your archetypal roles, pay attention to how they affect you. See the parts of them that are healthy for you and the parts that are unhealthy. Identify where you hold on to old archetypal habits, and see where you could let go of the old habits and adopt new ones. It can be difficult to change the way you deal with your archetypes. It can be difficult to go against your tribe's beliefs about how an archetype should be lived. But it is vital for your health that you allow your archetypes to evolve into newer, healthier versions and let go of the old ones.

As you are working on identifying and evolving your archetypes, look back through history and remember the struggles of all the people who have lived before you. Especially in Western culture, people have worked tirelessly to create a world of personal freedom, a world where we all have the potential to manifest whatever our intuitions have drawn us to accomplish. In the past, people have given both their energy and their lives so we all could have that freedom. As you work to evolve your archetypal roles, you should consider it not only your right but also your responsibility to take advantage of the struggles of all the people who came before you. As you evolve your archetypes, you bring your own energy flow into healthy balance and you contribute to the evolution of our culture.

▶ *EXERCISE: Pay attention to your archetypes. Identify the different archetypes that you are living now and that you have lived in the past. Look at your work life, relationships with other people, personality traits, hobbies, and inner self to help you identify them.*

▶ *EXERCISE: Pay attention to how many energy units you currently put toward the activities, thoughts, and relationships associated with your different archetypes. How satisfied you are with the way you are living them? Are there aspects of the way you live your archetypes that you would like to change?*

▶ *EXERCISE: Identify any unhealthy intellectual messages you have associated with your archetypes. When you discover those messages, work to create healthy replacement messages. Also feel the emotions that come through you as you work with your archetypes. Finally, if you need to, change the way you live your archetypes. This will help bring your energy flow into healthy balance.*

▶ *EXERCISE: If you find an archetype you feel drawn to but have ignored, start investigating what you may be able to do to fulfill that archetype.*

The Mother Archetype

There are a few archetypes that are especially important to be aware of when you are working on healing yourself. One of these is the mother archetype. Every woman who has ever taken on the responsibility of nurturing and raising a child is living the mother archetype. It doesn't matter whether the child is her biological child, a foster child, or adopted. When she takes on the job of caring for that child, a woman becomes a mother.

The experience of being a mother is one of the most intense and powerful experiences a woman can have. The mother archetype requires women to make significant energy commitments to their children. Being a mother can be a miraculous and beautiful experience, but it can also be brutal and punishing. Mothers have traditionally been given almost total responsibility for taking care of their children's needs. While fathers have been expected to provide financial support, mothers have been responsible for all the hands-on care of their children. They have been responsible for their children's physical, emotional, and mental health. They have been responsible for their children's success and happiness. Mothers are responsible for keeping their young children safe, clean, well fed, and comfortable, but their responsibility doesn't end when a child is eighteen. Throughout their lives, children continue to depend on their mothers for support of all types.

The job of being a mother is unlike other jobs because mothers are always on call. Even when a mother takes a vacation and leaves her children with a trusted baby-sitter, she worries about her children. When her children are grown, live thousands of miles away, and have children of their own, a mother still worries about them. From the moment a woman becomes a mother until the day she dies, a woman lives the mother archetype. Even if a woman's child dies before she does, she never loses the feeling that she is a mother.

Mothers feel compelled to do everything in their power to take care of their children, even when they themselves are exhausted. A mother may have a severe energy deficit, and she may feel that she has nothing left to give, but she will dig deep down inside herself and give whatever she can find. She will accept the fact that she is making herself sick if that is what it takes to nurture her child.

Because of the responsibility that culture has placed on the mother archetype, children have a tendency to blame their mothers for everything that goes wrong in their lives. They blame their mothers for their unhappiness, bad habits, lack of success, and everything else under the sun. A person can be eighty years old, and her mother may have been dead for forty years, but she will still be blaming her mother for what went wrong in her life.

There is a big discrepancy between the responsibilities of the mother archetype and those of the father archetype. While mothers are expected to accomplish the world for their children, fathers have been given quite a different list of expectations. Fathers have traditionally been expected to provide two things: sperm and financial support for their children. Fathers have been considered to be too busy doing important things out in the world to help take care of children.

While the father archetype has been evolving, there is still a large chasm between our expectations for mothers and fathers. If a father abandons his children, people may think his behavior is bad, but there is nowhere near the stigma that there is when a mother abandons her children. After ignoring his children for many years, a father can come back and tell them that he'd like to get to know them now. The children may be angry but will often accept him back into their lives. It is a lot harder for children to forgive their mothers after similar abandonment. This is because the expectations for the mother archetype are so much greater than they are for the father archetype.

Fathers have become much more involved with their children in recent decades, but there is still a long way to go before the responsibilities of the mother and father archetypes become equal. When a father is highly involved in caring for his children, people still have a tendency to talk about what a wonderful father he is, as though it's really amazing that he would choose to take such an active role in his children's lives. When a mother is providing the same level of care for her children, people don't even blink because they expect a mother to always be highly involved in her children's care.

Being a mother can be a terribly unforgiving experience. Culture teaches mothers that they can't rest or be happy until everyone else in their lives is happy. Since that will never happen, mothers are essentially taught that it is never okay to rest or be happy. Mothers are frequently stuck in a state of constant hypervigilance. They have trouble relaxing and taking care of themselves. They feel shame if they shift their focus from their children to themselves.

Unfortunately, with the movement in recent decades of women into the workforce, the stress on women has doubled. Now they have to fulfill their mother archetypal roles *and* their career roles. It is as though they have to live two lives in one body. Finding a healthy balance between their mothering and their careers would be easier if they had enough support from the people around them. But many working mothers have poor support or none at all. Any mother who has a job and also does the majority of the child care, cooking, and household chores for her family is going to end up having an energy deficit. If a mother is chronically running on an energy deficit, she will eventually get sick.

Mothers are frequently trying to live up to impossible ideals. They want to make their children's lives perfect, yet they are living in imperfect situations with limitations on what they can accomplish. They may have financial problems that limit their ability to provide perfect lives for their children. They may have a partner who is unsupportive or abusive. There are a thousand things that can work against a mother's ability to make her children's lives perfect. Even the most perfect mother in the most perfect situation will still make mistakes.

Mothers need to be aware that they are living the mother archetype, and they need to acknowledge the great pressures that this archetype places on them. Of course every mother wants to do her best for her children. And as with all other archetypes, you should do your best to be true to the mother archetype. But you also need to recognize that there needs to be balance while you are living the mother archetype. Abusing yourself to take care of your children will bring your energy out of balance and will eventually take a toll on not only you, but also your family, when you get sick.

Mothers need to recognize when they have internalized unhealthy intellectual messages that are hurting them. They have to work to evolve those messages and the mother archetype into something healthier and more regenerative. For example, if a tribal message tells a mother that she doesn't deserve to rest until everyone else in her world is happy, she needs to work on letting go of that message. A replacement message may be: *If you sacrifice your health and your inner peace for the good of everyone around you, eventually you will have nothing more to give to yourself or anyone else. Eventually you will end up being a drain on everyone else's energy because they will have to take care of you when you get sick.*

Another tribal message that mothers commonly internalize is the idea that they are responsible for the success and happiness of their children. While it is true that the mother archetype requires mothers to do their best to help their children, mothers can't control how things are going to turn out for their children. We are all on this earth to learn life lessons, and it would be unrealistic to expect that anyone would have a perfect life with no pain and no challenges. When you try to control your children's lives and make them perfect, you are trying to go against the laws of nature. You are also interfering in your children's rights to learn the rich life lessons they need to learn.

Mothers are currently taught that they can and should do it all. But this isn't a realistic expectation to sustain for extended periods of time unless they have enough support from the other people in their lives. No one can do it all for very long without developing an energy imbalance. If doing it all starts to take a toll on you and makes you exhausted and physically sick, there is a problem.

You can't be the best mother that you can be if you are sick and exhausted. You can't be true to the mother archetype if you let yourself get out of balance.

If you are a mother and find yourself getting physically and emotionally exhausted, you need to work to bring your energy into balance. Of course there are going to be days when you have to give more than your one hundred energy units for your family, but if this is happening on a chronic basis, you need to recognize that it is happening and work on healing the system.

As you are working on living the mother archetype in a healthy way, think about the emergency oxygen-mask instructions that flight attendants give passengers at the beginning of a flight. They tell parents that in an emergency, they should put their own oxygen masks on first and then put their children's masks on. This is so that parents will have enough oxygen to survive and take care of their children. How much good are you to your child if you give her the oxygen mask first but don't have enough time to put on your own mask? What if because of your lack of oxygen, you die during the emergency? Your child may die, even with her oxygen mask on, because you aren't there to care for her during the crisis.

The same issue comes up for mothers in everyday life, although the situations are not usually so dramatic. If you are giving all your oxygen and energy to your children and the other people in your life, eventually you will get depleted. Although you may want to be the caretaker, in the end you won't be able to take of anyone else if you don't take care of yourself first.

The most responsible thing a mother can do for herself and her family is to find balance in her life. You need to take care of yourself in order to have the energy to take care of the people you love. This concept of self-care is much more involved than simply taking a bubble bath once in a while. You need to use your intuition to figure out how to prioritize where you are going to spend your one hundred energy units every day.

It is your responsibility to figure out what you need and to follow through and get it. This involves every aspect of your life. You need to know what you have to do to take care of your body. How much rest do you need? What diet is right for you? How much exercise do you need? You need to know what you have to do to take care of your relationships. Who are you going to spend your time with? How much time are you going to spend with them? You need to know what you have to do to take care of other aspects of your life. Is your job situation the right one for you? Is there another archetype that is also important to you? It may be hard to make the necessary changes to bring things into balance. It may take time and energy to identify what you need and figure out how to follow through with it.

As you are working on finding balance in your life, it is imperative for you to remember that your children have their own dramas to experience. It can be easy to want to jump in and take over directing the action in your children's dramas. Mothers tend to want to turn their children's dramas from intense dramas with a lot of action to boring shows that are no more exciting than watching paint dry. For a mother, the more boring her children's dramas are, the better.

As children grow up, there is only going to be one way for them to learn how to make healthy decisions for themselves. That is by testing themselves, taking risks, and seeing how things turn out. If you are a mother who is watching your children make decisions that you judge as bad or if you are watching them feel deep emotions, you can't interfere in their dramas. You need to step back, feel your emotions, and try not to judge the situation. Nothing annoys and alienates your children more than being judged and controlled. And you don't have the energy units to waste.

It is also important to remember the mother archetype as you look at your relationship with your own mother. Every mother does the best she can. Some mothers disappoint their children by making small mistakes, and some do unspeakable things that traumatize their children for life. As difficult as it can be to accept the things your mother has done, in order to heal yourself, you cannot judge your own mother any more than you can judge yourself for your mothering.

Everyone makes mistakes, and some people make terribly harmful choices, mothers included. All mothers do the best they can with the resources they have. Your mother's best may be judged as terrible, but still it is the best she could do in the situation. This is why it is so important to remember the concept that we are all here on this earth to learn life lessons. If a mother makes a mistake and her child ends up having a painful lesson to learn because of that mistake, neither the mother nor the child can judge that experience. As with all dramas, the experience must be grieved and work must be done to heal unhealthy intellectual messages. But to hold on to a judgment about why the mother is so terrible is not helpful for her child's energy flow any more than it is for the mother's energy flow.

▶*EXERCISE: If you are a mother (or someone who isn't actually a mother but tends to feel overly responsible for taking care of other people as mothers do) start watching for your mother archetype and pay attention to the unhealthy intellectual messages you have associated with it. Do the work needed to calm those unhealthy intellectual messages, and feel the emotions you have connected to your mother archetype. Take action and make any changes you need to in order to live your mother archetype in a healthier way.*

The Macho-Man Archetype

The macho-man archetype is experienced by most men. They may not realize that it is affecting them, but it is. When we think of the macho man, we may think of the Clint Eastwood type: men who are strong, silent, and in control. Or we may think of loud, pushy bullies who are aggressively protecting their territory. But you don't have to be as dramatic as the stereotypical macho men in the movies to live the macho-man archetype. Most men end up living this archetype whether they recognize it or not.

The driving motivation for the macho-man archetype is the ability to control emotions. Throughout history, men have been expected to be tough and strong. They had to kill the bears and drag them home for their wives to cook over their fires. They were expected to protect their families from the warriors in the neighboring tribes. They were taught that they always had to be in control. They could never let down their guard because if they did, their tribe may perish.

Men have learned that if they are going to be strong and in control, they can't feel their emotions. They've been taught that it is a sign of weakness to feel most emotions. Fear and sadness are considered the most dangerous emotions because they expose a man's vulnerability. And even feeling too much joy can be a sign of weakness. The only emotion that they are taught is acceptable is anger, but they don't learn to feel their anger in a healthy way. Instead, they learn to project their anger onto the people around them and yell and scream and make dramas, and that is very unhealthy.

Although culture is evolving and men don't have to drag the bear carcass home anymore, they are still holding on to many of the old intellectual messages associated with the macho-man archetype. They are still holding on to the unhealthy messages they've been given about emotions. They continue to try to keep their happy masks (or maybe in this case they are angry masks) plastered firmly in place, and they continue having trouble letting anyone see their vulnerability, including their wives and families.

The problem with the macho-man archetype is that it is not healthy. While men have physically dominated over women for thousands of years and they seem to have had all the power, they have paid a huge price for that power. When you can't feel your emotions, you can't find warmth or comfort inside yourself. When you are constantly focused on your intellectual messages, life takes on a cold hard sense of reality and there is little spontaneity or magic.

When you can't feel emotions or show your vulnerability, you can't have healthy relationships with other people. And the imbalance between your emotions and your intellect brings your energy out of balance. Although men have had much physical and financial power, they've ended up paying the price for that power in the loss of their inner peace.

Currently there is somewhat of a shift occurring in our culture regarding men and emotions. It is becoming more acceptable for men to feel their emotions. But there is still a blatant discrepancy in the way boys and girls are raised. Boys are treated differently, starting when they are babies. Little boys are still expected to be strong and fit the macho-man archetype. If a little boy is crying over something considered too girlish, the adults around him do what they can to get him to buck up and be a man. As much as people give lip service to letting boys feel their emotions, most parents are still uncomfortable with this.

As boys grow older, the macho-man archetype is reinforced from every direction. Parents, teachers, and other children are constantly giving them feedback to let them know if they are being too feminine or too emotional. While young men today may not be as obviously macho as men from older generations, this is still a problem. Boys and younger men continue to put a significant amount of their energy units every day into blocking their emotions.

To heal themselves, men need to recognize and work to heal the unhealthy intellectual messages associated with this archetype. The predominant unhealthy message is the one that tells you that it is weak to feel emotions and that you always have to be tough and strong. Depending on your particular tribes, you may have learned other unhealthy messages about the macho-man archetype as well. You may have learned that men need to be good athletes or smart or successful in business to be "real" men.

You need to work on calming the unhealthy intellectual messages associated with the macho-man archetype. Step back and observe yourself and other men you know, and try to see the situation from a new perspective. See that the strongest and most courageous thing a man can do is feel his emotions. Because everyone is so afraid of doing it, you have to be very courageous to do it. Practice feeling your emotions, and learn how to experience them in a healthy way. Remember that you don't have to feel your emotions in public or make yourself vulnerable, but at some time during your day, you have to allow your emotions to flow in order to have healthy energy flow.

And finally, follow your intuition as it guides you to know other things you need to do to evolve the macho-man archetype. Do you need to change the way you relate to other people? Do you have to stop being so competitive? Take the action steps needed for you to be able to relax and enjoy being a man instead of always having to live up to an outdated archetype.

It is important for women to recognize the macho-man archetype in the men in their lives. Many conflicts between men and women stem from the macho-man archetype. An area where this is especially true is with emotions. Women will often recognize when the men in their lives are having trouble feeling their emotions. A woman may notice that her man is acting more sullen and withdrawn or angrier than usual.

Women will try to help by trying to get their men to talk about their emotions. But the last thing that people who are suppressing their emotions will want to do is talk about them. When you try to get a macho man to talk about his emotions, he will get uncomfortable and may withdraw further or may project his anger toward you. This creates an unhealthy drama.

For example, a man's father may die, and he may have a lot of grief to feel over the loss of his father. But he may not be able to feel the grief because he has learned that sadness is weak. Because he can't feel his sadness, it builds up in his emotional organ. If there is a lot of grief building up inside him, he may have to work hard to keep it from spewing out. The actions that he takes to hold the lid on the emotional organ closed may end up being unhealthy and dramatic. He may start drinking excessively or doing drugs so he doesn't have to feel his emotions. He may take up a solitary hobby, such as running or hunting, that allows him to isolate himself from other people. He may find other ways to withdraw from the people who are close to him. Occasionally his emotions might push their way out of his emotional organ, and he may channel his grief into another emotion, such as anger. He may end up projecting his anger onto his family, and he may get mad at little things that have nothing to do with his original grief.

It is important for women to recognize when their men's macho-man archetypes are making it difficult to resolve a conflict. If you are a woman in this situation, step back and take a different approach. If you try to get a macho man to talk about his feelings or work through a conflict when he isn't ready, you will just waste your energy and make him angrier. Instead of trying to solve the conflict by changing yourself or changing him, step back and let him be. Do your own work on the drama. Feel your emotions. Do your work with the mirror, and recognize any unhealthy intellectual messages he is mirroring for you. Work on your side of the conflict until you understand your part in it.

Then when you are ready, use your intuition to help you know what the most advantageous step will be for you. You may want to talk to the macho man at a time when you are both feeling neutral and less emotional. If the conflict centers on his problem with suppressing his emotions, you may want to tell him that you think he needs to work on feeling his emotions. You may tell him how he is hurting your relationship by putting all his energy into blocking his emotions rather than using it for more regenerative activities.

As you are talking to him, remember that you can't change him unless he is ready to change. You can't make him feel his emotions if he isn't ready to. You can't make him do any other things he doesn't want to do. Your purpose for talking to him is to let him know what you need from him so that you can resolve the conflict together. Your purpose in talking to him is not to change him or fix him.

Hopefully he will be willing to work with you. But if he decides he doesn't want to deal with his emotions or whatever else you requested of him, you ultimately have two options: accept your man the way he is or let him go. What you decide to do will depend on what your intuition guides you to do. It depends on how much energy the relationship is taking from you and whether it is worth it—energywise and healthwise—to stay. But whatever you choose, don't waste any more of your energy trying to talk him into being something he doesn't want to be.

▶EXERCISE: *If you are a man (or a woman who identifies with the macho-man archetype), you will want to investigate your life for the macho-man archetype. Pay close attention to your relationship with your emotions. Pay attention to your reaction to other people when they feel their emotions. Macho men are uncomfortable with emotions. It doesn't matter how nice or how gentle you appear. If you won't let yourself feel your emotions, you are experiencing the macho-man archetype.*

▶EXERCISE: *Work with the macho-man archetype the way you would work with any other archetype. Look at unhealthy intellectual messages you have internalized from your tribes that reinforce the macho-man archetype. Work on evolving those messages. Feel your emotions. Finally, make the necessary changes to evolve your macho-man archetype into a new, healthier version.*

▶EXCERICE: *If you are a woman who is dealing with a macho man, pull your energy back from him and do your work on your side of the drama. Feel your emotions. Use him to mirror any unhealthy messages you have inside yourself and heal those messages. Finally, take the action step that your intuition guides you to take, and remember to stop wasting your valuable energy units trying to change him if he doesn't want to change.*

The Patient Archetype

The patient archetype is experienced by people who are either physically or mentally ill. When you are sick, you frequently aren't able to live life the way you did when you were well. Maybe you have lost your normal physical function, or maybe you can't do the social activities you used to enjoy. The degree to which your life has changed will determine how strongly your life is affected by your patient archetype.

When you are a patient, you can feel terribly frustrated. If you can't do the things you want to do, you can feel as though you've lost your identity. Many people who are living the patient archetype are searching for a way to heal themselves and get their lives back as close to normal again as possible. They can be highly motivated to do what they need to do to heal, but they can also get depressed and hopeless and feel paralyzed by the situation.

The patient archetype can take over every aspect of your life. If you don't feel well, every activity you do and every interaction you have can be affected. Your entire perspective toward life can change. What you previously took for granted takes new significance. Little things, such as being able to clean your house, take a walk, or play with your grandchildren, may now be a challenge.

Patients develop a variety of symptoms, depending on their specific illness. These symptoms can be very exhausting and require a lot of energy to manage. For example, if you have chronic pain or fatigue, you may need to rest more than you did in the past. You may find yourself becoming more intensely focused on yourself than you did when you were well. You may not have the same level of energy you used to have. You may have to pull some of your energy units back from your relationships and the activities you used to do and use them to take care of your body. This can be hard on your relationships with your family and friends. They may be hurt or angry because of the way that you have changed. They can withdraw from you, and this can make you feel more isolated and depressed.

If you find that your patient archetype is a significant archetype for you, you will want to work with it to learn the lessons it has to teach you. As with the other archetypes, you will want to identify and heal any unhealthy intellectual messages associated with it. And you will want to feel the emotions the archetype triggers.

There is some work that is needed for the patient archetype to evolve in our culture. Patients have traditionally learned to take a very passive approach toward health and healing. People in our culture have a tendency to neglect and abuse their bodies with the assumption that if they get sick, their physicians will come through with a strong treatment to make them better. In response, physicians have learned to take on an authoritarian and paternalistic role toward their patients; they hand their patients a prescription or recommend a surgery with an attitude that says, *My child, I know all the answers. Just depend on my judgment. I know this will heal you.* Western medicine is very powerful at treating acute conditions, and it can also be effective at controlling many chronic ones. So people assume that when they get sick, there will always be a quick fix to heal them.

The problem comes when the physician's treatments don't work. At that point your approach to your patient archetype needs to evolve. The new patient archetype requires that you, the patient, recognize the power you have over your own healing. This doesn't mean you should stop going to your physician. Patients should continue to use their physicians as experts to help them when they need medications or surgical procedures. And if you find that alternative-medicine therapies are effective for you, you should continue using them as well. But you also need to take one hundred percent responsibility for the healing you can do for yourself.

As you work on evolving your patient archetype, try to start seeing your healing from a different perspective. Instead of seeing illness as a problem that just begins and ends in your body, recognize that your healing requires that all areas of your life be in balance. Ask yourself where the imbalances are.

As you are looking for the places in your life where there are imbalances, you can look at your body and observe how well you are taking care of it. Listen to what your intuition has to say about the situation.

If you find something that needs to change, change it. But if you find that your energy is too far out of balance for you to effectively make the change, put the physical change aside for the time being and focus on bringing your energy system into balance. What is going on with your energy flow? Is it out of balance? Pay attention to the symptoms in your body to help you know if your energy is flowing in a healthy way or not.

To bring your energy flow into healthy balance, work on both sides of the emotion/intellect balance. Open up your emotional organ and feel your emotions. Recognize when shame is blocking your healthy emotional flow, and work to let go of the judgments behind the shame. Work on calming your intellect, and use your dramas to learn the lessons they have to teach you. Make the changes in your life that your intuition guides you to make. Identify your life lessons, and do the work needed to take your energy units back from any unresolved issues connected with them. Recognize your archetypes, and do any work that is needed to evolve them into healthier versions of the old archetypes.

The work of healing yourself can be difficult at times. You may need to rest when you are feeling your deep emotions, especially in the beginning as you start to clean out your emotional basement. You may need to be disciplined as you start to identify your unhealthy intellectual messages and work on letting them go. You may also find that there are significant changes you need to make in your life in order to heal. Maybe you will need to change jobs or leave a relationship. Your intuition will guide you to let you know what will be the most beneficial thing for you to do.

It can take some time to bring your energy system back into balance. Remember that you have lived with your old habits for your entire lifetime. Don't expect to change the situation in a few days or weeks. Try to have patience as you are doing your work. Remember that our physical bodies are part of nature. Nature frequently works on a different time schedule than our intellects would like. Your intellect may think that things should be moving along faster than they are. But if your body and your energy system have work to do, you can't force things to progress faster than they are meant to go. Trust that your system will come into balance in the right time, and you will find yourself feeling better—emotionally and physically.

As you are feeling more energy, you can start to focus on the physical issues, such as diet, exercise, and other physical changes. Listen to what your body and your intuition are telling you about what you need. Each of our bodies has its own specific needs. We each have a specific diet that our body prefers. We also have our own specific needs for exercise and rest. It is your job as a patient to figure out what you need to do to be healthy and apply your energy units to the change.

The patient archetype can be a difficult archetype to work with. No one wants to be sick. No one wants to lose their normal function. But instead of letting your patient archetype make you hopeless and depressed, try to see it as a life lesson that can help you learn about yourself and learn about healing.

▶ *EXERCISE: If you are experiencing the patient archetype, look at the intellectual messages you have associated with it. Look at your expectations of your physicians and of yourself. If you have unhealthy intellectual messages, such as those that tell you can't heal yourself, work with your intellect to adopt healthy replacement messages. Feel the emotions triggered by your patient archetype. Listen to your intuition as it guides you to know what you need to do to take care of yourself.*

The Victim Archetype
The victim archetype is the part of us that feels vulnerable, like a victim. It is activated when we are in situations where the outcome appears to be out of our control. It is also activated when we think another person has power over us. Our victim archetype makes us feel trapped, hopeless, and depressed.

We all have times in our lives when our victim archetype becomes activated. When you have an illness, you can feel like a victim because you can't control what is happening to your body. If your company downsizes and you lose your job, you can feel like a victim of the economy. If you can't make it home for Christmas because of a bad storm, you may feel like a victim of Mother Nature.

Our victim archetype also gets activated in dramas in which we feel that someone else is taking advantage of us. If your neighbor stole your doll when you were five years old, you may have felt victimized by her. If your employer pays you less than you think you should be paid, you may feel victimized by your employer. If your spouse makes promises and doesn't follow through, you may feel victimized by your spouse.

We all have a victim archetype. We all have times in our lives when things seem to be out of our control. We all have times when we feel vulnerable. The problem with the victim archetype is that because it is associated with a sense of vulnerability and loss of control, people are frequently ashamed of it. When you are ashamed of being a victim, it is hard to face it and work through it.

As you are working on healing yourself, it will be your job to recognize your victim archetype. You will want to see your victim archetype not as a shameful thing to hide, but as another life lesson to learn from. You will want to evolve your approach to your victim archetype the same way you evolve your other archetypes.

To recognize your victim archetype, pay attention to past or present situations in which you have felt like a victim. Look at your dramas and identify situations in which you have felt hurt, abused, or trapped. If you are feeling shame about a situation in which you are vulnerable, your victim archetype may be involved. If you are feeling anger or sadness because you think you are being treated unfairly, you may be experiencing the victim archetype. If you are feeling fear because the outcome of a situation is unknown or because someone has threatened you, you may be experiencing the victim archetype.

Another way of recognizing times when you feel like a victim is to watch the way you interact with other people. If you find yourself making passive-aggressive comments toward other people, you will want to figure out why. Are you making those comments because you feel angry about being victimized? It can be tempting to deal with your sense of victimization by projecting your anger onto other people as a way to protect yourself.

Once you have identified your victim archetype, you will want to work on healing it. The victim archetype is like shame; you will want to identify it, but you don't want to live in the state of victimization forever. When you feel like a victim, it can be easy to get stuck in a state of paralysis, and when you are stuck in the victim archetype, you block your energy flow.

To heal your victim archetype, you will want to work on both sides of the emotion/intellect balance and bring them into balance again. First you will want to feel your emotions. Feel all the anger, fear, and sadness you need to feel about the situations that activate your victim archetype. Don't tell yourself that you shouldn't be angry or hurt or afraid over a certain situation that makes you feel like a victim. Every victim situation—big or small—needs to be processed emotionally.

You will also want to work on the intellect side of the balance and identify and calm any unhealthy intellectual messages associated with your victim archetype. To do this you will want to separate the situations that activate your victim archetype into two categories: impersonal situations that involve your loss of control over your life, and dramas that make you feel like a victim of other people. The first category includes all the situations in which you are experiencing painful life lessons that aren't any one person's doing. For example, if you are sick or your child is sick, it may not be any one person's fault. You may feel trapped and victimized by the situation, but there may not be anybody who can change the details of the situation. The second category includes situations in which you feel victimized by other people. They may actually be doing something to victimize you, or you may simply be feeling victimized; either way, your sense of victimization needs to be dealt with.

You will find that the way you deal with the intellectual messages in the two categories will be slightly different. When you are dealing with the impersonal situations, it is easy to get stuck on the intellectual treadmill and focus on the details of how the situation is victimizing you. You may think about how it is so unfair that God is doing this to you. You may try to look back and ask yourself how you could have prevented this from happening. You may worry about how the future will turn out.

Instead of focusing on the details of how the situation is victimizing you, pull yourself away from the intellectual treadmill and see the bigger picture. Imagine that you are up in the hot-air balloon looking down on yourself, and see yourself acting out your drama. Then look down at all the houses on the street, and visualize the people in those houses as they are learning their own lessons too. Look into the windows and see them having dramas, emotions, and challenges of their own. Be aware that everyone on the earth is experiencing life lessons, and you are not the only one.

Recognize that it is a natural part of life to have challenging situations. We are on this earth to learn lessons, not just to have fun and look good. Try to see these life lessons not just as random acts of cruelty from God but as situations that are teaching us things we need to learn. We may not want to learn these lessons, but these lessons are the cost of doing business as human beings.

Also remember that everyone has a victim archetype. When you feel like a victim, you can feel very isolated and alone. But the truth is that everyone has situations in which they feel like a victim, no matter how successful, rich, strong, or beautiful they are. People may put on their happy masks and pretend that everything is always easy for them, but that is a lie. We all have times when our lives feel out of our control. If you recognize that being a victim is a universal experience, you won't need to think that you are so alone.

Remember that although you may end up in a situation you didn't choose, you always have control over the way you will deal with the outcome. You are one hundred percent responsible for the way you deal with every situation. If you choose to stay on the intellectual treadmill judging the situation, you can get stuck in a miserable outcome. But if you choose to feel your emotions and work on changing your intellectual messages and finding a new perspective about the situation, you may be able to change it in some way. For example, you may be feeling victimized because your car broke down and you don't have enough money to fix it. First, feel your emotions. Maybe you are angry about your car breaking down. Next, step back from the situation, and see it from a different perspective. Look down on it from the hot-air balloon. See that you aren't the only person who doesn't have a car. Many people can't afford to have a car. And as you are looking down on the situation from this new perspective, see your car breaking down as a reason to walk or ride a bike more. This may be better for your health and may allow you to meet more people in your neighborhood. The situation has now evolved into one in which you are in control of your destiny.

Not all situations can be changed. For example, if you are dealing with cancer, you may have no choice but to go through the cancer treatments if you are going to have a chance of surviving. In this situation, maybe the only thing you can change is the way you deal with it. You still need to feel your emotions. And although you may not be able to change the details of the situation, you can still change your perspective. As you step back and view the situation from a different point of view, you can see that many people get cancer. You are not alone. Remember that although this experience might be awful for you, it is a life lesson and we all have to live through our life lessons.

Try to be open to whatever this lesson is teaching you. Maybe the lesson is that you need to learn how to ask for support from the people around you. Maybe the lesson is that you need to learn how to stop and rest and feel your emotions. Maybe the lesson is that you have to learn to listen to what your body needs. The process of stepping back and viewing the situation as a life lesson will change the way you experience it. This will help you let go of your sense of victimization.

The other category of situations that activates your victim archetype includes the dramas in which you feel like a victim of other people. Dramas involving a victim and a victimizer are very common. Some of these dramas are very obvious and immediately recognizable. But in some situations the victimization is more subtle. This can be especially true if you have a close relationship with your victimizer. If you have had a long history together or if your lives are very closely entwined, it can be hard to step back and see the truth about the situation.

Victimization can be subconscious, even for the victimizer. Victimizers may appear to be nice and caring, and they may not consciously realize they are being victimizers. They may be friendly and sociable and interested in being a part of your life. Your victimizer can simultaneously hurt you and want to be close to you. This can make the victim/victimizer drama confusing.

People often start playing the roles of victim and victimizer when they are children. We tend to fall into habits regarding what role we will play. Some people always end up being the victim, and some people always end up being a victimizer. People frequently play both roles, depending on the situation. You may be the victim in some relationships and the victimizer in others.

Once you have recognized that you are involved in a victim/victimizer drama, you will want to start by feeling all the emotions it triggers. You will also want to work with the intellectual messages associated with being a victim. Victims tend to feel trapped and controlled by their victimizers. It can seem that the victimizers have all the power in the drama and the victims have none.

You will want to change your perspective toward the victim/victimizer drama. Start by stepping back and viewing it from a historical perspective. Human beings have been competing for survival for thousands of years, so we've gotten into the habit of thinking there always has to be a winner and a loser, a victimizer and a victim. This has been a habit for so long that even in our modern Western culture we continue to perpetuate it, although we don't have to.

Billions of victim/victimizer dramas have been acted out throughout history. And if you could look, at this moment, into all the houses and businesses in the world, you'd see millions of victim/victimizer dramas being acted out while you read this book. It's as though the victim/victimizer drama is one of the most popular shows in television history, and the television executives keep ordering more shows every season because we just can't get enough of them.

See how you and your victimizer are acting out an archetypal drama that started thousands of years ago. Acknowledge that you've been taught your part in the drama by your culture. Your tribes, through the intellectual messages they taught you, conditioned you to be a victim. See how your victimizer has also learned his or her part from the culture. Try to see how interchangeable your victim/victimizer drama is with the millions of other similar dramas being acted out around the world every day. Recognize that much of what you have learned about your part in the drama is simply habit and can be changed.

When you are involved in a victim/victimizer drama, it can be easy to take everything very personally. It can be easy to get caught up in the drama and feel that the victimizer is doing bad things to you only because of qualities in you that are weak or inadequate. It can be easy to look at your victimizer as a monster who victimizes you simply because he or she is such a terrible person. Try now to see that although this drama feels very personal, you are both acting out your parts using the victim/victimizer script that has been around for thousands of years. Try to see things as not being so personal. When you see the drama with this perspective, hopefully it will lose some of its hold over you.

When you are observing the victim/victimizer drama, step back and observe the different ways that people react to the drama. Sometimes people try to find a reason for why they are being victimized. An abused spouse may try to explain why her abuser continues to hurt her. She may tell a friend, "He just lost control; he didn't really mean to hit me. I really made him angry. It's my fault that he hurt me." She is using her intellect to tell a story to explain the situation. Even though her intuition is telling her to get out of the situation before she gets killed, her intellect is keeping her trapped in the situation with the stories it is telling.

Some people who are being victimized dissociate from the reality of the situation. Children and adults who have been severely traumatized may be so stressed by a dangerous situation that they suppress their memory of the experience. Because of the dissociation, they may not recognize that they have been victimized. The problem with this approach is that the memory of the trauma is still in their bodies. Although they don't remember what happened, they are still being affected by it. Over time this can lead to both mental and physical illness. And if they don't acknowledge and work through their victim archetype, they may be more vulnerable to being victimized again in the future.

Some people who are victimized feel a deep sense of shame. Because tribal messages tell us that to be vulnerable is a shameful thing, it is common for victims to deny, to themselves and others, that they are being victimized. An example of this is a child who is being bullied at school. The child is experiencing the victim archetype, but he has learned the message that being a victim is a shameful thing. He may not tell his parents or teachers about the bullying because he knows he will be seen as a weak, vulnerable victim. He may think that his father will tell him to face the bully and fight back, but he may not feel comfortable doing that. Or he may think that the adults will tell him to just ignore the bully, but he knows that isn't possible. A child in this situation may feel trapped and ashamed, and because of the shame he won't be able to work to find a healthy resolution to the situation.

Some victims respond to a situation of victimization with anger. They may realize immediately that they have been victimized, and they may be tempted to confront their victimizer. They may project their anger toward their victimizer, either aggressively or more subtly. They may become violent because they don't know how to feel their anger in a healthy way. Or instead of being overtly angry, they may act out their anger with passive-aggressive behaviors. This can create more drama and be potentially dangerous. This approach can also cause them to perpetuate the victim/victimizer drama instead of working on getting to the root of the problem.

Some people have learned to deal with their victim archetype by victimizing others. They are uncomfortable with the sense of vulnerability that accompanies the victim archetype. They don't want to admit to themselves that they feel like a victim; instead, they have figured out that one way of avoiding that feeling of vulnerability is to become a victimizer. They find someone else to hurt, and they victimize that person. They say or do things they know will hurt the other person.

The problem with this approach is that although a victimizer may avoid feeling like a victim for a little while, in the end the sense of being a victim is still inside him or her. If a teenage boy is being abused by his father, he may learn to deal with his sense of victimization by becoming an abuser as well. When he is feeling vulnerable and his victim archetype is triggered, he may start acting out and hitting his girlfriend as a way to feel less vulnerable. But the problem is that, in addition to feeling like a victim himself, he has now hurt his girlfriend and made her a victim too. By victimizing his girlfriend, he has brought more pain and shame into his life.

Whenever people are cruel or deliberately take advantage of other people, you can be sure that deep inside they really feel like victims themselves. They may seem tough and mean on the outside, but on the inside they are feeling vulnerable. And while it may be hard to see from the outside, a victimizer wastes a lot of energy units on his or her efforts to hurt others. It may not be obvious immediately, but over time victimizers pay a huge price—energetically and physically—for their actions.

Whenever you are feeling victimized by another person, use your knowledge about the victim archetype to change your perspective toward the situation. Remind yourself that the person who is victimizing you feels like a victim too. You may not be able to see the victimizer's sense of vulnerability, but you can trust that it is there. Remember that people who are at peace with the world don't need to victimize others.

Your goal in seeing your victimizer as a vulnerable person is not so that you will feel sorry for your victimizer. Feeling sorry for other people is based on the judgment that they are weak or pathetic. Remember that judgments are not healthy, and pitying people because of a judgment you make about them is not healthy. Feeling sorry for your victimizer makes you tempted to allow the victimization to continue, and that isn't healthy. When you feel sorry for your victimizer, you may make excuses for the victimizing behavior. You may think, *My poor abuser is so pathetic that I can't blame him or her for abusing me and I'll overlook the abuse.* That will not break the victim/victimizer cycle.

Your goal in seeing your victimizer as vulnerable is so that you can see that that person isn't more powerful than you are. Even though the other person may seem to currently have more power in the situation, he or she is human just as you are. Your victimizer is your equal, not more powerful than you and not less powerful than you. He or she may have control of the outcome in this specific situation, but you are still equal.

As you work on shifting your perspective toward your victimizer, feel the emotions that are triggered. You will find that as you work on both sides of the emotion/intellect balance, you will start to let go of your sense of victimization. You will also start to hear your intuition more easily. Your intuition will help you know what will be the most beneficial thing for you to do to resolve the situation and break the victim/victimizer cycle.

The victim archetype is a powerful archetype that affects us all. It is a major cause of distress for many people. Whether you feel like a victim because of a painful life lesson that is out of your control or because you are involved in a victim/victimizer drama, your victim archetype needs to be addressed. Only when you identify your sense of victimization can you work through it and heal it. It can take courage to face your victim archetype because of the shame it may bring, but true healing cannot be accomplished without facing this part of your inner self.

▶ EXERCISE: Identify situations in which your victim archetype has been activated. You can recognize your victim archetype in situations in which you have felt hurt, used, abused, or taken advantage of. Let yourself feel all the emotions triggered by your victim archetype.

If you have shame over being a victim, look at the intellectual messages at the root of your shame. Is it because you feel weak and vulnerable when you are a victim? Or is there another message that triggered the shame for you?

Work on developing new intellectual messages to replace the unhealthy messages associated with your victim archetype. If you are in a situation that appears to be out of your control, remember that everyone has a victim archetype and that the situations that are out of our control are situations that teach us valuable life lessons, no matter how painful they are. Remember that you are not alone in experiencing the victim archetype.

If you are feeling victimized by another person, see how that person also has a victim archetype and is no less vulnerable than you are. Remember that no one who is feeling a sense of inner peace will want to victimize another person, so obviously your victimizer must feel like a victim too, if he or she is victimizing you. Also step back and see how the victim/victimizer drama is a historical one that you don't have to perpetuate.

Finally, listen to your intuition as it guides you to make the changes you need to make to resolve the situation.

▶ EXERCISE: Pay attention to the people around you, and recognize their victim archetypes and the situations in which they appear to feel and act like victims. This will help you see that we all have a victim archetype, and we all have times when we are a victim or feel like a victim.

▶ EXERCISE: Look at the victim archetype from the other side of the drama. See a situation in which you have taken the part of the victimizer *in the historical victim/victimizer drama. See how somewhere inside you was the sense of victimization that caused you to react by victimizing someone else. Feel the emotions triggered as you recognize what you have done, and work on finding new healthier intellectual messages to replace the message that tells you to victimize other people. Finally, take the action steps you need to take to stop victimizing others.*

The Addict Archetype

The addict archetype is experienced by people with addictions. The type of addiction doesn't matter; as long as you have an addiction, you are experiencing the addict archetype. It can be hard to recognize that you have an addiction, and it can be harder to let go of that addiction once you recognize you have it. To bring your energy flow into healthy balance, you need to work on healing your addictions.

We frequently think of addiction in the context of abuse of substances, such as drugs and alcohol. And while these substances can be especially unhealthy and dangerous when they are abused, they are by no means the only things you can become addicted to. There are many other addictions that can harm you.

Almost everyone in our culture has an addiction of some type. To identify your addictions, you can start by using substance addictions as an example to help you understand what makes a habit an addiction. When people are addicted to a substance, they develop a compulsive physical and psychological craving and need for it. Their need for the substance drives addicts to put their use of it ahead of other aspects of their lives. They ruin their relationships, lose their jobs, and get into financial and legal trouble because of their inability to control their use of the substance.

There are many people who use habit-forming substances and do not become addicted. They may use these substances for entertainment or for medical reasons, and they are able to use them without losing control. Unfortunately, some people find that their use of a particular substance spirals out of control. They use more than recommended, and they use the substance to manage their emotions and stress instead of just using it for its original purpose. Their lack of control escalates until their use of the substance becomes the central concern in their lives. And because of the characteristics of habit-forming substances, people who become addicted to them have to deal not only with the emotional aspects of being addicted but also with the strong physical cravings that develop when their bodies get dependent on these substances.

There are many other habits and behaviors that can get out of control the same way that the use of substances can. You may start doing these things for entertainment or as a basic lifestyle habit, but over time you may do them as a way to deal with the stress in your life. As you do them more frequently, you can lose control over them and they can become addictions that can take over your life. Any habit or behavior can be considered an addiction if it has gotten out of control to the point that it is harmful for you and is very difficult to stop. Some of these behaviors are called obsessions or compulsions instead of being called addictions.

Some examples of addictions that start out as nonaddictive activities include shopping, gambling, and sex. If your shopping or gambling gets so out of control that it ruins your finances, it is hurting you. If your sexual habits become compulsive to the point that they ruin your relationships or endanger your health, they are hurting you. When you lose your ability to control these activities and they are hurting you, you have an addiction to them.

Another common addiction is the compulsion to eat too much food. Many food addicts start using food to comfort themselves in times of stress or to deal with suppressed emotions. As they get more dependent on food to manage their emotions, they have a harder time controlling their eating and they gain weight.

There are other habits that can develop into addictions. Work can turn into an addiction. If you work such long hours that your spouse leaves you or you don't have time to exercise or take care of your body, you are harming yourself. The problem with an addiction like workaholism is that it is culturally sanctioned, and workaholics are actually rewarded for their addiction. This can make it difficult to recognize that your workaholism is a problem.

Another common addiction is perfectionism. If you always need to be perfect or look perfect or have things in your life be perfect, you are a perfectionist. Individual perfectionists have different criteria regarding what they consider important. Some need to keep a clean house. Some need to do a perfect job at work. Some need to always dress the right way. Perfectionism is based on your particular judgments about what is right and what is wrong.

Perfectionism, like workaholism, is another addiction that our culture rewards. If you are a perfectionist, you can be very successful at work or at whatever you decide is important to you. People may look at you and try to emulate your perfect ways. It can be very addicting to keep up your perfect image. The problem with perfectionism, as with all other addictions, comes when you harm yourself with your efforts to be perfect. If you ruin relationships because of your unrealistic expectations of yourself or other people, your perfectionism is harming you. If you can't relax or you make yourself sick because your intellect is busy pushing you to be perfect, your perfectionism is harming you.

Addictions usually start when people are young, in their teens and early twenties. At the root of many addictions is the inner conflict that is created when people's emotions and intellects get out of balance. As children lose the ability to feel their emotions, they lose their connection to their natural way of being. They lose their ability to soothe themselves during times of stress. They also lose the ability to listen to their intuitions and figure out what they need to do in order to take care of themselves and feel safe and secure.

As their intellects become more judgmental, their lives start to feel cold and hard. The magic of childhood is lost and replaced by shame. The feeling of shame and the process of shutting off their connection to their inner selves can create a chasm deep inside them that is so uncomfortable that they try to find something to help them escape from it. They need something to help them find that feeling of warmth and security again, so they start looking outside themselves to whatever habits or behaviors are most comforting for them. Everyone is drawn to something different; some people are drawn to substances, some are drawn to addictive behaviors, and some are drawn to both.

The problem with addictions is that they can limit you from doing the work you need to do to heal yourself. As you put your energy units into the activities required from your addictions, you take those energy units away from healthy, regenerative activities. Addictions also interfere with the healthy function of both sides of the emotion/intellect balance. Your addiction keeps the lid on your emotional organ tightly closed. When you do feel your emotions, the flow is affected. It can either be blunted or it can become dramatic and out of control. If you allow your emotions to build to intense levels before they burst out of your emotional organ, you can easily project your emotions onto the people around you in unhealthy or dangerous ways.

Addictions also affect the intellect side of the emotion/intellect balance. If you are addicted to a substance, the substance can limit your cognitive clarity. This will make it difficult to recognize and change your unhealthy intellectual habits. If you are addicted to a behavior, your intellect can get so strongly stuck on the thought treadmill as it focuses on the behavior that it can be difficult to pull yourself away from the treadmill and observe yourself. This will make it hard do the work of calming your intellect.

It is important to recognize your addictions. Be honest with yourself. If you find yourself having trouble controlling a habit that is affecting you in an unhealthy way, it is possible that it is an addiction. If you are having trouble deciding whether it is an addiction, ask people who you trust what they think. Sometimes you need help from someone else if your addiction is clouding your insight. Also listen to your intuition. Deep inside you is the voice that knows the truth regarding whether a certain habit is unhealthy for you. Your intellect may have trouble accepting that it is an addiction, but your intuition knows the truth.

Part of the reason why it is hard for people to face their addictions is that addictions often have a sense of stigmatization associated with them. Tribes make many judgments against addicts. It can be hard to admit to yourself and to other people that you have an addiction if your tribe makes a judgment that addicts are bad. The judgment against you can cause you to feel shame about your addiction, and this will make you want to keep it a secret.

When you are dealing with your addictions, it is important for you to remember that almost everyone has some type of addiction. No type of addiction is better or worse than the others. The different addictions all have their own special constellation of lessons that come with them. If you aren't lucky enough to have a culturally sanctioned addiction, such as workaholism or perfectionism, remind yourself not to judge your specific addiction, even if other people do. Remind yourself that the only way you will be able to heal yourself is to acknowledge and work through your addiction.

▶*EXERCISE: Identify your addict archetype and the addiction behind it. Be honest with yourself about what your addiction is. Pay attention to whether you feel a sense of shame about your addiction, and investigate the judgments behind the shame. Work with both sides of the emotion/intellect balance: feel your emotions while you work to find healthy replacement messages to replace shameful ones.*

▶*EXERCISE: If you have an addiction to a substance, such as a recreational drug or a prescription drug, that you can't stop using on your own, get professional help to stop using it. You also may need help to stop unhealthy behaviors such as gambling or sex addiction. As you are working on healing your addiction, apply the concepts in this book. When you have cravings for the substance or behavior, feel the emotions that are triggered instead of trying to dull them with the substance or behavior.*

Work to identify and heal unhealthy intellectual messages that are hurting you. And work with the other aspects of your life that need healing, including your dramas and other life lessons.

▶ EXERCISE: *If you have a food addiction, make a healthy diet plan. When you are craving food that is unhealthy for you or having trouble controlling the amount of food you are consuming, pay attention to what you are feeling and let yourself feel it instead of using the food to suppress the emotion. Identify and calm the unhealthy intellectual messages that may be contributing to your drive to overeat.*

If you find that you don't have enough energy to change your diet immediately, do your inner work and leave the details of the diet in the background for a while. Later on, as you bring your energy into balance, you can come back to your diet and apply your energy units to making the changes needed.

▶ EXERCISE: *If you are a perfectionist or a workaholic, identify the areas in your life where you are especially controlling and driven, then deliberately limit activities in those areas. For example, if your drive to have a spotless house is interfering with your relationship with your family because you are always arguing with them about keeping it clean, force yourself to let things get messy. Deliberately leave dishes in the sink overnight, and leave your children's toys scattered in the living room. As you sit and look at the mess and feel agitated, let yourself feel the emotions that are triggered. Also look for underlying judgments that may be driving your addiction (for example,* I am a bad wife and mother if I have a messy house*), and work on letting go of those judgments.*

9 Conclusion

The job of healing yourself is not always an easy one. It can take time, energy, and diligence to look into all the areas of your life that are out of balance. It can be hard to face the parts of yourself that aren't so pretty. It can be hard to take one hundred percent responsibility for every aspect of your healing and your life. But only when you view your life with this perspective can you truly heal yourself.

As you are working on healing yourself, expand your concept of health to involve not only your physical body but also your underlying energy flow. Incorporate your new understanding of energy flow into your everyday thoughts, so you can make this new concept real for yourself. Pay attention to where you are spending your energy units every day. Make it your goal to pull your energy units back from your unhealthy thoughts and activities and to use them instead for healing and regenerative activities.

Develop a healthy balance between your emotions and your intellect. Be aware of how those two parts of you are totally separate, and be able to identify the way they interact with each other. Open the lid on your emotional organ and let your emotions flow. Don't just tell yourself, *I know that everything will be okay, so I don't need to be emotional.* Instead, tell yourself, *Everything may turn out all right, but I still have emotions to feel, and I know that in order to be healthy, I need to feel them.* Recognize that the key to having healthy energy flow is to allow your emotions to flow.

Watch your intellect as it gets stuck on the intellectual treadmill, and work on both sides of the emotion/intellect balance to calm the unhealthy intellectual habits that are wasting your energy units. Identify your tribes and the unhealthy intellectual messages they have taught you. Remember that no tribal message is worth holding on to if it doesn't support your individual health. Remember that you are your own best expert and that you know better than anyone else what is most beneficial for you.

Watch yourself as you live out your dramas, and use every drama, no matter how big or small, to help you understand yourself better. See your dramas not as conflicts that are making you stressed out but as situations that are there to teach you lessons about yourself. Use your dramas to unearth the emotions you need to feel, and use them as mirrors to help you identify unhealthy intellectual messages that need healing. Also use your dramas to help you identify the changes you need to make in your life.

Be aware of your archetypes so you can live them in a healthy way. Be aware of when you are letting old tribal approaches to your archetypes hurt you, and evolve them into newer healthier versions of the old archetypes. When painful life lessons activate your victim archetype, allow yourself to feel the emotions they trigger and remember that you aren't alone in your pain. We all have life lessons to learn, and it's much healthier to face those lessons and heal them rather than to put on a happy mask and avoid them.

Finally, listen to your intuition as it gives you guidance about the path that is most beneficial for your life. Let your intuition drive your car, and let your intellect step out of the driver's seat and into its role as the GPS. As you calm your intellect and feel your emotions, your intuitive voice will become easier to hear. You will be able to use your intuitive guidance to know what you should do regarding your physical health and other issues in your life. You can then use your emotional flow as the fuel for your car's trip through life.

CONCLUSION

Applying these new ideas takes time. It takes time to stop and feel your deep emotions. It takes time to identify your unhealthy intellectual messages. It takes time to understand how the other aspects of your life are affecting your health. The beauty of this process is that at its root is the goal of returning to your natural way of being, the way you lived when you were a young child. So although changing your perspective may be difficult in the beginning, once you start to experience the changes in your energy and your health, your new habits will be natural and easy to maintain over time.

One aspect of this work that can be especially difficult is when what you need to do goes against what the other people in your life want you to do. But no matter what other people think, you need to make the changes that are right for you to get your energy flowing in the healthiest way possible. If you don't make the changes and you continue to allow yourself to be hurt by situations that are unhealthy, you will continue to feel physically ill and lack inner peace.

Ultimately every person is responsible for the way his or her life unfolds. We are all one hundred percent responsible for our own healing. Your physicians can do their part, but they can't heal everything. You are the only one who can identify and heal the aspects of your inner life that are out of balance. The work you do to bring your energy flow into balance will be the work that will heal your physical body and bring you inner peace.